MCQs for FRCS

DATE DUE

14.5.13	
7/10/13	
3/9/15	

GAYLORD   PRINTED IN U.S.A.

Examination Collection

MCQs for FRCS

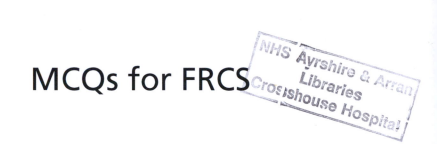

SOMAIAH AROORI
Senior Clinical Fellow in Transplant Surgery
Addenbrooke's Hospital, Cambridge

AND

DR PUNEET
Ex-Surgical Fellow
Liver Unit, Queen Elizabeth Hospital, Birmingham

Radcliffe Publishing
London • New York

Radcliffe Publishing Ltd
33–41 Dallington Street
London
EC1V 0BB
United Kingdom

www.radcliffepublishing.com
Electronic catalogue and worldwide online ordering facility.

British Library Cataloguing in Publication Data

A catalogue record for this book is available from the British Library.

ISBN-13: 978 184619 493 1

The paper used for the text pages of this book is FSC® certified. FSC (The Forest Stewardship Council®) is an international network to promote responsible management of the world's forests.

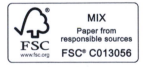

MIX
Paper from
responsible sources
FSC® C013056
www.fsc.org

Typeset by Pindar NZ, Auckland, New Zealand
Printed and bound by TJI Digital, Padstow, Cornwall, UK

Contents

Preface

This MCQ book for the FRCS General Surgery exit examination is designed to meet the needs of higher surgical trainees preparing for the Part 1 exit exam. The FRCS exit examination is the final hurdle that surgical trainees have to pass before they can be given the green light to apply for the Certificate of Completion of Training. The curriculum for the General Surgery exit examination is extensive and it is essential to have a broad knowledge of general surgery and other surgical sub-specialisations, e.g. breast, endocrine, oesophagogastric, hepatobiliary, etc., in order to pass the exit exam. We know a lot of trainees who failed the Part 1 exam several times due to lack of knowledge in areas other than their chosen sub-specialties. At the time of my [SA] preparation for the exit examination, I could not find a single MCQ book that was aimed at the higher surgical trainee which covered the entire intercollegiate surgical curriculum. This led us to write this book comprising MCQs covering the entire surgical curriculum except for medical statistics.

This book covers all areas of general surgery and sub-specialties, including emergency surgery, and the questions are organised according to sub-specialty. The complexity of questions varies from specialty to specialty and in some chapters there are questions on applied anatomy, physiology and the fundamentals of surgery while in others there are more clinically-based questions. Where possible, we have ensured that there are no controversial questions and multiple or ambiguous answers. We strongly recommend that trainees read the relevant subject material before attempting to answer the questions in any particular area. We hope that this book will help trainees to focus on the areas they need to concentrate on and learn more about a particular topic. It will also be useful not only with preparation for Part 1 but also for the viva component of the exit and MRCS examinations due to the extensive coverage of the relevant clinical topics and applied anatomy, physiology and critical care. The book is also of relevance for trainees preparing for the exit examination in other surgical specialties who require some knowledge of general surgery.

We wish good luck and success to every surgical trainee in their career.

Somaiah Aroori
Puneet
January 2011

About the authors

Somaiah Aroori graduated from Guntur Medical College, Guntur, Andhra Pradesh, India in 1995. He is the winner of several gold medals including gold medal for the best outgoing student of University of Health Sciences, Andhra Pradesh, India. He undertook his postgraduation (MS) in general surgery at the most prestigious institution in India, the All India Institute of Medical Sciences, New Delhi. He came to the UK in 1999 for higher surgical training in general surgery. He did two years of cancer research and was awarded Doctor of Medicine (MD) in 2005 from Queen's University of Belfast. He received his national training number in general surgery in August 2004 and started training at Derriford Hospital, Plymouth. He has a special interest in teaching and was awarded the post-graduate certificate in medical education from Peninsula Medical School in 2009. He completed his FRCS General Surgery exit examination in February 2009 and was awarded the Certificate of Completion of Training (CCT) in July 2010. He is currently working as a Senior Clinical Fellow in Transplant Surgery at Addenbrooke's Hospital, Cambridge.

Puneet graduated from the Institute of Medical Sciences, Banaras Hindu University, India in 1995 and undertook his postgraduation (MS) from the same University in 1998. He then worked as a senior registrar in Ram Manohar Lohia Hospital, New Delhi in India for 3 years. In 2003, he was appointed as Assistant Professor of Surgery at the Institute of Medical Sciences, Banaras Hindu University, Varanasi. He has presented several papers at conferences, published more than 40 national and international papers and written six chapters in books. He worked as a Surgical Fellow in the Liver Unit, Queen Elizabeth Hospital, Birmingham in 2009–10. He was made a Fellow of the American College of Surgeons in 2010.

Acknowledgements

I am eternally grateful to my friend Dr George Laycock for her support throughout the preparation of this book. In particular, however, I am eternally grateful to Dr Puneet for making this book possible and without whose motivation and support this book would not have been possible. I am grateful to my wife Sreevidya and my daughters Saahi and Saanvii for putting up with my prolonged absences.

Somaiah Aroori
January 2011

1
Endocrine
surgery

Questions

1. C-cells in the thyroid gland are derived from:
   a Neural crest.
   b Ultimobronchial body.
   c Thyroglossal duct.
   d Fourth pharyngeal pouch.

2. Which of the following statements regarding venous drainage of the thyroid gland is incorrect?
   a The middle thyroid vein drains into the brachiocephalic vein.
   b The superior thyroid vein drains into the internal jugular vein.
   c The inferior thyroid vein drains into the brachiocephalic vein.
   d None of the above.

3. The superior thyroid artery is closely related to the following nerve:
   a Recurrent laryngeal nerve.
   b Hypoglossal nerve.
   c External laryngeal nerve.
   d Glossopharyngeal nerve.

4. The recurrent laryngeal nerve is closely related to:
   a Superior thyroid artery.
   b Inferior thyroid artery.
   c Thyrocervical trunk.
   d Middle thyroid artery.

5. The most common location of a thyroglossal cyst is:
   a Subhyoid.
   b Over the thyroid cartilage.
   c Suprahyoid.
   d Sublingual.

6. The complications associated with thyroglossal cyst include all of the following, except:
   a Abscess formation.
   b Thyroglossal sinus/fistula.
   c Malignancy.
   d Thyrotoxicosis.

7. Graves's disease is due to:
   a Hypersecretion of thyroid stimulating hormone.
   b Abnormal thyroid stimulating antibodies.
   c Anti-mitochondrial antibodies.
   d Increased secretion of thyroxine.

8. Which of the following features is not associated with primary thyrotoxicosis?
   a Goitre is diffuse and vascular.
   b Exophthalmos is more common.
   c Cardiac failure is more common.
   d None of the above.

9. The treatment of choice for a 35-year-old pregnant female with thyrotoxicosis is:
   a Radioactive iodine.
   b Anti-thyroid drugs.
   c Surgery.
   d β-blocker.

10. The preferred treatment of choice in a child with thyrotoxicosis is:
    a Radioactive iodine.
    b Subtotal thyroidectomy.
    c Total thyroidectomy.
    d Anti-thyroid drugs.

11. The most common cause of hypercalcaemic crisis is:
    a Carcinoma of the breast.
    b Parathyroid hyperplasia.
    c Parathyroid adenoma.
    d Paget's disease.

12. The anti-thyroid drug of choice in the pre-operative preparation of a thyrotoxicosis patient is:
    a Lugol's iodine.
    b Carbimazole.
    c Propanolol.
    d Propylthiouracil.

✓ 13. Iodide alone is not used in the pre-operative preparation of a thyro-toxicosis patient because:
    a It can make thyrotoxicosis worse.
    b It can increase the vascularity of goitre.
    c Rapid control of thyrotoxicosis is not possible.
    d None of the above.

14. Which of the following statements regarding the use of β-blockers in the pre-operative preparation of thyrotoxic patients is incorrect?
    a It acts rapidly.
    b It abolishes the clinical manifestations of sympathetic over-activity.
    c It inhibits the peripheral conversion of T4 to T3.
    d It should be stopped just after surgery.

15. The reason why the inferior thyroid artery is not routinely ligated during thyroidectomy is:
    a To avoid injury to the recurrent laryngeal nerve.
    b To avoid injury to the external laryngeal nerve.
    c To preserve the blood supply to the parathyroid glands.
    d To avoid injury to the parathyroid glands.

16. The thyroid cancer that originates from C-cells is:
    a Follicular carcinoma.
    b Papillary carcinoma.
    c Medullary carcinoma.
    d Anaplastic carcinoma.

17. The most common type of thyroid cancer in females is:
    a Follicular carcinoma.
    b Papillary carcinoma.
    c Medullary carcinoma.
    d Anaplastic carcinoma.

18. The thyroid cancer that is associated with multiple endocrine neoplasia (MEN) is:
    a Follicular carcinoma.
    b Papillary carcinoma.
    c Medullary carcinoma.
    d Anaplastic carcinoma.

19. Which of the following groups of patients with papillary thyroid cancer have the worst prognosis?
    a Women aged 50 and younger.
    b Older patients with tumour <5 cm.
    c Patients with intrathyroid papillary carcinoma.
    d Patients with distant metastasis.

20. The superior parathyroid gland develops from:
    a Third parapharyngeal pouch.
    b Ultimobronchial body.
    c Fourth pharyngeal pouch.
    d Sixth pharyngeal pouch.

21. Which of the following statements is incorrect regarding the embryology of the inferior parathyroid glands:
    a They develop from the third pharyngeal pouch.
    b They have a short pathway of descent.
    c Their location varies widely compared to the superior parathyroid glands.
    d 50% of inferior parathyroid glands are located in the vicinity of the inferior thyroid pole.

22. All of the following are functions of parathyroid hormone, except:
    a It increases the serum calcium level by increasing the absorption of calcium from the kidneys.
    b It helps in the hydroxylation of 25-hydroxycholecalciferol to 1,25 dihydroxycholecalciferol.
    c It inhibits renal tubular secretion of phosphate and bicarbonate.
    d It increases serum calcium levels by increasing the turnover of bone.

23. The hormone that is a physiological antagonist to parathyroid hormone is:
    a   Calcitonin.
    b   Thyroxine.
    c   1,25 dihydroxycholecalciferol.
    d   Glucocorticoids.

24. The most common symptom associated with hyperparathyroidism is:
    a   Fatigue.
    b   Abdominal pain.
    c   Constipation.
    d   Hypertension.

25. The treatment of choice in a patient with normocalcaemic hyperparathyroidism is:
    a   Calcium supplementation.
    b   Parathyroidectomy.
    c   Treatment with calcineurin.
    d   Administration of 1,25 dihydroxycholecalciferol.

26. A 45-year-old female patient presents with acute confusion, abdominal pain, vomiting and dehydration. Electrocardiogram shows prolonged P interval and shortened QT interval. The most likely electrolyte abnormality is:
    a   Hypercalcaemia.
    b   Hypomagnesaemia.
    c   Hypocalcaemia.
    d   Hyponatraemia.

27. The common cause of hypercalcaemia in non-hospitalised patients is:
    a   Primary hyperparathyroidism.
    b   Malignancy.
    c   Iatrogenic.
    d   Milk alkali syndrome.

28. The diuretic used in the first-line treatment of hypercalcaemia is:
    a   Furosemide.
    b   Spironolactone.
    c   Bendroflumethiazide.
    d   None of the above.

29. The agent used as second-line therapy in the treatment of hypercalcaemia is:
   a   Loop diuretics.
   b   Pamidronate.
   c   Calcitonin.
   d   Glucocorticoid.

30. The most common cause of primary hyperthyroidism is:
   a   Single parathyroid adenoma.
   b   Multiple parathyroid adenomas.
   c   Parathyroid hyperplasia.
   d   Parathyroid carcinoma.

31. The most sensitive and specific imaging method for the localisation of a parathyroid adenoma is:
   a   CT of the neck.
   b   Magnetic resonance imaging (MRI) of neck and chest.
   c   Thallium technetium pertechnetate scan.
   d   Sestamibi scan.

32. Which one of the following statements regarding sestamibi scan is incorrect?
   a   Sestamibi is a derivative of technetium.
   b   The large number of mitochondria in a hyperactive gland allows intense labelling with sestamibi.
   c   It is highly sensitive and specific in the localisation of parathyroid adenoma following previous parathyroid surgery.
   d   It is associated with a low dose of radiation and high-definition imaging.

33. The imaging method useful in the localisation of recurrent primary hyperparathyroidism following previous surgery is:
   a   Magnetic resonance imaging (MRI).
   b   CT scan.
   c   Ultrasound.
   d   Sestamibi scan.

34. All of the following features will help in the differentiation of parathyroid carcinoma from parathyroid adenoma, except:
    a Presence of palpable mass.
    b Presence of high serum calcium levels.
    c Involvement of recurrent laryngeal nerve.
    d Distant metastasis.

35. The most common cause of secondary hyperparathyroidism is:
    a Chronic renal failure.
    b Rickets.
    c Osteoporosis.
    d Hypermagnesaemia.

36. Secondary hyperparathyroidism is associated with:
    a Hypocalcaemia and hypophosphataemia.
    b Decreased bony resistance to PTH.
    c Decreased synthesis of calcitriol.
    d None of the above.

37. Indications for parathyroidectomy in secondary hyperparathyroidism are:
    a Failed medical treatment.
    b Intractable bony pain.
    c Asymptomatic ectopic calcification.
    d a and b.

38. Which of the following statements regarding tertiary hyperparathyroidism is incorrect?
    a It resolves spontaneously in over 60% of cases.
    b It is due to antibody production against parathyroid hormone (PTH).
    c Surgery is only indicated for persistent hypercalcaemia after 12 months of observation.
    d It is usually seen in patients with chronic renal failure after kidney transplantation.

39. The anatomical landmark useful in the localisation of the superior parathyroid gland is:
    a External laryngeal nerve.
    b Most cranial branch of the inferior thyroid artery.
    c Recurrent laryngeal nerve.
    d Inferior cornu of the thyroid cartilage.

40. The second most common location of the inferior parathyroid gland is:
     a Along the thyrothymic ligament.
     b Just behind the inferior pole of the thyroid gland.
     c Retrotracheal.
     d Retro-oesophageal.

41. After initial bilateral exploration of the neck for the parathyroid glands, a further search should not be continued if:
     a No gland or fewer than four glands have been discovered and none is pathological.
     b All four glands have been discovered and one or more are abnormal.
     c Fewer than four glands are discovered and at least two are enlarged.
     d All four glands are discovered and are normal.

42. Which one of the following statements regarding multiple endocrine neoplasia (MEN)-IIa syndrome is incorrect?
     a Primary hyperparathyroidism associated with MEN-IIa is more aggressive than in MEN-I.
     b The majority of patients with MEN-IIa often have multiglandular disease.
     c Aggressive resection of the parathyroid gland is not recommended.
     d Phaeochromocytoma should be excluded before treating hyperparathyroidism.

43. The follow-up of patients with parathyroid carcinoma is mainly done by:
     a CT scan of the neck.
     b Measuring serum calcium.
     c Measuring calcitonin.
     d Ultrasound of the neck.

44. Which of the following group of patients have the highest incidence of hypercalcaemia following parathyroidectomy?
     a Primary hyperparathyroidism due to adenoma.
     b Primary hyperparathyroidism due to multiglandular hyperplasia.
     c Familial hyperparathyroidism.
     d Patients with normocalcaemic hyperparathyroidism.

45. The main risk of parathyroid surgery in a patient with multiple endocrine neoplasia (MEN)-IIa is:
    a   Hypoparathyroidism.
    b   Recurrent laryngeal nerve injury.
    c   Hypercalcaemia.
    d   Recurrence of symptoms.

46. The superior thyroid artery is a branch of the:
    a   Thyrocervical trunk.
    b   External carotid artery.
    c   Internal carotid artery.
    d   Brachiocephalic trunk.

47. The inferior thyroid artery is a branch of the:
    a   External carotid artery.
    b   Thyrocervical trunk.
    c   Internal carotid artery.
    d   Brachiocephalic trunk.

48. Thyroid stimulating hormone (TSH) is released from the:
    a   Posterior pituitary gland.
    b   Thalamus.
    c   Hypothalamus.
    d   Anterior pituitary gland.

49. The metabolic effect of thyroid hormone is exerted mainly by:
    a   Free T3 and T4.
    b   Free T4.
    c   Free T3.
    d   Bound T4.

50. Serum thyroxine binding protein is increased with all of the following, except:
    a   Nephrotic syndrome.
    b   Pregnancy.
    c   Oral contraceptive pills.
    d   Oestrogens.

51. Medullary thyroid cancer is associated with germline mutations of which of the following oncogenes:
    a   RET proto-oncogene.
    b   K-ras oncogene.
    c   C-erb.
    d   ABL.

52. Iodine radioisotope scanning is not useful in the:
    a   Diagnosis of medullary thyroid carcinoma.
    b   Diagnosis of a solitary toxic nodule.
    c   Diagnosis of toxic multinodular goitre (MNG).
    d   Localisation of ectopic thyroid tissue.

53. Follicular carcinoma can be differentiated from follicular adenoma by:
    a   Presence of capsular invasion.
    b   Presence of vascular invasion.
    c   Presence of mitotic figures.
    d   a and b.

54. Which one of the following statements regarding the anatomy of the recurrent laryngeal nerve is incorrect?
    a   It curves around the sixth aortic arch on the left side.
    b   It curves around the subclavian artery on the right side.
    c   A non-recurrent laryngeal nerve is nearly always observed on the right side.
    d   It is a branch of the glossopharyngeal nerve.

55. Which one of the following statements regarding follicular carcinoma is incorrect?
    a   It is the second most common thyroid cancer.
    b   Previous irradiation of the neck is a risk factor.
    c   It is more common in females.
    d   It spreads mainly via the lymphatics.

56. All the following are characteristic features of follicular carcinoma, except:
a It commonly affects females.
b Fine-needle aspiration cytology is associated with high sensitivity and specificity for the diagnosis of follicular carcinoma.
c Hürthle cell variant is associated with a greater propensity for multifocality.
d Lymph node involvement is rare.

57. Which one of the following factors does not affect the prognosis of well-differentiated thyroid cancer?
a Age of the patient.
b Grade of the tumour.
c Extent and size of the tumour.
d Lymph node involvement.

58. The treatment of choice in a patient with well-differentiated thyroid cancer is:
a Total thyroidectomy.
b Subtotal thyroidectomy.
c Total thyroidectomy and modified neck dissection.
d Hemi-thyroidectomy and berry picking of lymph nodes.

59. The most common presentation of well-differentiated thyroid cancer is:
a Dominant nodule in a multinodular goitre.
b Solitary thyroid nodule.
c Solitary palpable cervical lymph node.
d Screening ultrasound of neck.

60. The marker that is useful for detecting recurrence of a well-differentiated thyroid cancer is:
a Free T3.
b Thyroglobulin.
c Bound T3.
d Calcitonin.

61. I^{131} scan is useful in the detection of metastatic disease following total thyroidectomy in all of the following thyroid cancers, except:
a Papillary cancer.
b Follicular cancer.
c Minimally invasive follicular carcinoma.
d Hürthle cell tumour.

62. Which of the following statements regarding medullary thyroid cancer (MTC) is incorrect?
   a It is an autosomal dominant condition.
   b 80% of the cases are familial.
   c It originates from parafollicular cells.
   d Calcitonin is used as a tumour marker.

63. Medullary thyroid cancer (MTC) associated with worst prognosis is:
   a MTC associated with MEN-IIa syndrome.
   b MTC associated with MEN-IIb syndrome.
   c Sporadic MTC.
   d b and c.

64. Which of the following statements regarding anaplastic carcinoma is incorrect?
   a Prognosis is frequently poor.
   b Surgical resection is possible in most of the patients.
   c Peak incidence is between 60–70 years of age.
   d Involvement of the surrounding structures is common.

65. A 25-year-old female presents with an acute painful thyroid swelling associated with malaise and fever following a recent sore throat. The most likely diagnosis is:
   a Acute thyroiditis.
   b Sub-acute thyroiditis.
   c Autoimmune thyroiditis.
   d Riedel's thyroiditis.

66. On histological examination, psammoma bodies are found in:
   a Follicular carcinoma.
   b Anaplastic carcinoma.
   c Papillary carcinoma.
   d Medullary carcinoma.

67. The type of thyroiditis that is associated with a high risk of lymphoma of the thyroid gland is:
   a Sub-acute thyroiditis.
   b Riedel's thyroiditis.
   c Hashimoto's thyroiditis.
   d Acute suppurative thyroiditis.

68. Damage to which of the following nerves results in a change in the pitch, range and projection of the voice?
    a External branch of superficial laryngeal nerve.
    b Recurrent laryngeal nerve.
    c Internal laryngeal nerve.
    d Glossopharyngeal nerve.

69. The external superficial laryngeal nerve is most likely to get damaged during:
    a Ligation and division of the middle thyroid vein.
    b Ligation and division of the inferior thyroid vein.
    c Ligation and division of the superior thyroid vessels.
    d Separation of the thyroid isthmus from the trachea.

70. Glucocorticoids are mainly produced by which layer of the adrenal cortex?
    a Zona glomerulosa.
    b Zona fasciculata.
    c Zona recticularis.
    d All of the above.

71. The most common cause of Cushing's syndrome is:
    a Adrenal adenoma.
    b Iatrogenic.
    c Pituitary adenoma.
    d Ectopic ACTH producing tumours.

72. All of the following changes occur in primary adrenal hyperplasia, except:
    a Hypokalaemia.
    b Hyponatraemia.
    c Hypernatraemia.
    d Water retention.

73. Conn's syndrome is associated with all of the following features, except:
    a Hypertension.
    b Muscle weakness.
    c Hypokalaemia.
    d Oedema.

74. All of the following are features of Cushing's syndrome, except:
     a Hypoglycaemia.
     b Hypertension.
     c Psychosis.
     d Hypokalaemia.

75. A high prevalence of skin pigmentation, muscle weakness and hypokalaemia is associated with which type of Cushing's syndrome?
     a Ectopic secretion of ACTH.
     b ACTH secreting pituitary adenomas.
     c Adrenal adenoma.
     d Iatrogenic.

76. Which of the following tests is helpful in the differentiation of Cushing's syndrome due to pituitary tumours or due to an ectopic source of ACTH?
     a 24-hour urinary cortisol.
     b Elevated midnight serum cortisol level.
     c Low-dose dexamethasone suppression test.
     d High-dose dexamethasone suppression test.

77. Hyperpigmentation following bilateral adrenalectomy is due to:
     a Hypersecretion of ACTH.
     b Iatrogenic long-term use of steroids.
     c Adrenal failure.
     d None of the above.

78. Which of the following statements regarding adrenal carcinoma is incorrect?
     a It is associated with a poor prognosis.
     b Most of them are non-functional.
     c It is usually >5 cm.
     d It is associated with MEN-I syndrome.

79. Which of the following agents is used in the treatment of adrenal carcinoma?
     a Mitotane.
     b Doxorubicin.
     c Flucanozole.
     d Mitomycin.

80. Most phaeochromocytomas are:
    a Malignant.
    b Benign.
    c Bilateral.
    d Extra-adrenal in origin.

81. Phaeochromocytomas can be associated with:
    a Multiple endocrine neoplasia syndrome.
    b Von Recklinghausen's disease.
    c Von Hippel–Lindau syndrome.
    d All of the above.

82. Which of the following statements regarding phaeochromocytomas is incorrect?
    a Extra-adrenal tumours are more common in children.
    b Most of them are familial.
    c Malignancy is more common in extra-adrenal tumours.
    d It originates from chromaffin tissue.

83. Phaeochromocytomas commonly present with:
    a Hypertension.
    b Heart failure.
    c Arrhythmias.
    d Myocardial ischaemia.

84. Hypertension associated with phaeochromocytoma should be treated with:
    a α-blockers.
    b α-blockers followed by β-blockers.
    c β-blockers.
    d β-blockers followed by α-blockers.

85. The radioactive isotope scan useful in the localisation of phaeochromocytoma is:
    a Metaiodobenzylguanidine (MIBG) scan.
    b Technetium pertechnetate scan.
    c Sestamibi scan.
    d I^{131} scan.

86. A 35-year-old female is diagnosed with phaeochromocytoma during the second trimester of pregnancy. The most appropriate treatment in this patient is:
    a Laparoscopic adrenalectomy during the second trimester.
    b α-blockers followed by caesarean section with or without synchronous adrenalectomy.
    c α-blockage followed by vaginal delivery.
    d α-blockage followed by medical termination of pregnancy.

87. The most common cause of primary aldosteronism is:
    a Adrenal adenoma.
    b Bilateral micronodular hyperplasia of the adrenal gland.
    c Bilateral macronodular hyperplasia of the adrenal gland.
    d Adrenal cortical carcinoma.

88. Mineralocorticoids are secreted from the:
    a Zona glomerulosa.
    b Zona fasciculata.
    c Zona reticularis.
    d Adrenal medulla.

89. All of the following conditions can cause secondary hyperaldosteronism, except:
    a Chronic liver disease.
    b Cardiac failure.
    c Nephrotic syndrome.
    d Conn's syndrome.

90. Which of the following drugs must be stopped before performing assay for diagnosis of hyperaldosteronism?
    a Spironolactone.
    b Calcium-channel blocker.
    c Fluconazole.
    d Oral contraceptive pills.

91. The electrolyte abnormality associated with primary hyperaldosteronism is:
    a Hypokalaemia.
    b Hyperkalaemia.
    c Hyponatraemia.
    d Hypocalcaemia.

92. An 18-year-old male patient underwent bilateral adrenalectomy
    for bilateral phaeochromocytoma. 48 hours following surgery he is
    feeling very tired and lethargic. His blood pressure is 80/60 mmHg
    and his pulse rate 90/min. Clinical examination does not reveal any
    signs of volume loss. The most likely diagnosis is:
    a Sepsis.
    b Cardiogenic shock.
    c Addisonian crisis.
    d Hypovolaemic shock.

93. The most common tumours associated with multiple endocrine
    neoplasia (MEN)-I syndrome are:
    a Insulinomas.
    b Adrenal cortical tumours.
    c Pituitary tumours.
    d Parathyroid adenomas.

94. The majority of pancreatic islet tumours associated with multiple
    endocrine neoplasia (MEN)-I syndrome are:
    a Functional.
    b Non-functional.
    c Multicentric.
    d b and c.

95. The most common pituitary tumours associated with multiple
    endocrine neoplasia (MEN)-I syndrome are:
    a Prolactinomas.
    b ACTH secreting tumours.
    c Non-functioning pituitary adenomas.
    d Growth hormone secreting pituitary tumours.

96. All of the following tumours are associated with multiple endocrine
    neoplasia (MEN)-I syndrome, except:
    a Insulinomas.
    b Glucagonomas.
    c Gastrinomas.
    d Phaeochromocytomas.

97. Which one of the following features is associated with aggressive tumour behaviour in a patient with multiple endocrine neoplasia (MEN)-I associated gastrinoma:
   a Tumour size >3 cm.
   b Onset of gastrinoma at 50 years of age or older.
   c Diagnosis of MEN-I at 35 years of age or older.
   d Low level of gastrin at the time of presentation.

98. The treatment of choice for pituitary prolactinomas is:
   a Surgery.
   b Radiotherapy.
   c Surgery followed by radiotherapy.
   d Dopamine agonists.

99. Which one of the following statements regarding gastrinoma is incorrect?
   a Drug-induced achlorhydria can lead to false positive test results.
   b Proton pump inhibitors should be stopped 4 weeks before the measurement of serum gastrin levels.
   c All patients with gastrinomas should be tested for MEN-I syndrome.
   d Normal gastrin levels exclude the diagnosis of gastrinoma.

100. All of the following conditions are associated with MEN-II syndrome, except:
   a Hirschsprung's disease.
   b Medullary thyroid cancer.
   c Pituitary adenoma.
   d Phaeochromocytoma.

101. Genetic screening for germline RET mutations should be offered to:
   a New patients with two synchronous or metachronous features of MEN-II.
   b Patients presenting with medullary thyroid cancer.
   c Infants presenting with Hirschsprung's disease and family history of medullary thyroid cancer.
   d All of the above.

102. The majority of insulinomas are:
    a Benign and multiple.
    b Benign and extrapancreatic in origin.
    c Benign and solitary.
    d Extrapancreatic and multiple.

103. Addison's disease is characterised by all of the following features, except:
    a Hyperglycaemia.
    b Hypotension.
    c Hyperkalaemia.
    d Hyponatraemia.

104. The majority of carcinoid tumours originate from the:
    a Appendix.
    b Small bowel.
    c Colon.
    d Stomach.

105. Which one of the following statements regarding carcinoid tumours is incorrect?
    a All patients with jejunoileal carcinoids present with carcinoid syndrome.
    b The presence of carcinoid syndrome indicates liver metastases.
    c Patients with large retroperitoneal tumours can present with carcinoid syndrome.
    d Secretory diarrhoea is the most common feature.

106. A 25-year-old male patient presents with clinical features suggestive of acute appendicitis. At laparotomy he is found to have a 2.5 cm growth at the base of the appendix. He should be treated with:
    a Appendicectomy.
    b Right hemicolectomy.
    c Appendicectomy followed by right hemicolectomy at a later stage if the margins are positive.
    d Limited ileocaecal resection.

107. The treatment of choice for patients with rectal carcinoids of less than 1 cm size is:
    a Local excision.
    b Anterior resection.
    c Short-term chemotherapy followed by local excision.
    d Short course of radiotherapy followed by local excision.

108. Which one of the following statements regarding rectal carcinoids is correct?
    a Measurement of urinary 5-hydroxyindoleacetic acid (HIAA) is not useful.
    b Octreotide scan is very useful in the diagnosis of rectal carcinoids.
    c Tumours <2 cm have a high incidence of metastasis.
    d The lung is the most common site of metastases.

109. Which of the following imaging modalities is most sensitive for evaluation of an extra-adrenal phaeochromocytoma?
    a Ultrasound.
    b CT scan.
    c Magnetic resonance imaging (MRI).
    d Metaiodobenzylguanidine (MIBG) scan.

110. Phaeochromocytomas predominantly secrete:
    a Epinephrine.
    b Norepinephrine.
    c Dopamine.
    d Dihydroxyphenylalanine (DOPA).

111. Cushing's syndrome is not associated with which one of the following conditions?
    a Adrenal carcinoma.
    b Oat cell carcinoma of the lung.
    c Medulloblastoma.
    d Pituitary adenoma.

112. The metabolic abnormalities associated with hyperaldosteronism are:
    a Hypernatraemia, hypokalaemia, metabolic alkalosis.
    b Hyponatraemia, hypokalaemia, metabolic alkalosis.
    c Hyponatraemia, hyperkalaemia, metabolic alkalosis.
    d Hypernatraemia, hyperkalaemia, metabolic alkalosis.

113. The clinical features associated with Cushing's syndrome include:
     a Hirsutism.
     b Poor wound healing.
     c Bitemporal hemianopia.
     d All of the above.

114. The most common cause of Conn's syndrome is:
     a Adrenal adenoma.
     b Adrenal hyperplasia.
     c Adrenal carcinoma.
     d Liver failure.

115. The dominant clinical feature of Conn's syndrome is:
     a Generalised weakness.
     b Peripheral oedema.
     c Hypertension.
     d Polyuria.

116. The precursor for epinephrine and norepinephrine is:
     a Tyrosine.
     b Histidine.
     c Tryptophan.
     d Arginine.

117. Adrenaline and noradrenaline are the two most common hormones produced by the adrenal medulla. The ratio of these hormones is:
     a 2:1.
     b 4:1.
     c 1:8.
     d 1:6.

Answers: Endocrine surgery

1. a Neural crest.

2. a The middle thyroid vein drains into the brachiocephalic vein.

3. c External laryngeal nerve.

4. b Inferior thyroid artery.

5. a Subhyoid.

6. d Thyrotoxicosis.

7. b Abnormal thyroid stimulating antibodies.

8. c Cardiac failure is more common.

9. b Anti-thyroid drugs.

10. d Anti-thyroid drugs.

11. c Parathyroid adenoma.

12. b Carbimazole.

13. a It can make thyrotoxicosis worse.

14. d It should be stopped just after surgery.

15. c To preserve the blood supply to the parathyroid glands.

16. c Medullary carcinoma.

17. b Papillary carcinoma.

18. c Medullary carcinoma.

19. d Patients with distant metastasis.

20. c Fourth pharyngeal pouch.

21. b They have a short pathway of descent.

22. c It inhibits renal tubular secretion of phosphate and bicarbonate.

23. a Calcitonin.

24. a Fatigue.

25. b Parathyroidectomy.

26. a Hypercalcaemia.

27. a Primary hyperparathyroidism.

28. a Furosemide.

29. d Glucocorticoid.

30. a Single parathyroid adenoma.

31. d Sestamibi scan.

32. c It is highly sensitive and specific in the localisation of parathyroid adenoma following previous parathyroid surgery.

33. a Magnetic resonance imaging (MRI).

34. b Presence of high serum calcium levels.

35. a Chronic renal failure.

36. c Decreased synthesis of calcitriol.

37. d a and b.

38. b It is due to antibody production against parathyroid hormone (PTH).

39. a External laryngeal nerve.

40. a Along the thyrothymic ligament.

41. b All four glands have been discovered and one or more are abnormal.

42. a Primary hyperparathyroidism associated with MEN-IIa is more aggressive than in MEN-I.

43. b Measuring serum calcium.

44. c Familial hyperparathyroidism.

45. a Hypoparathyroidism.

46. b External carotid artery.

47. b Thyrocervical trunk.

48. d Anterior pituitary gland.

49. a Free T3 and T4.

50. a Nephrotic syndrome.

51. a RET proto-oncogene.

52. a Diagnosis of medullary thyroid carcinoma.

53. d a and b.

54. d It is a branch of the glossopharyngeal nerve.

55. d It spreads mainly via the lymphatics.

56. b Fine-needle aspiration cytology is associated with high sensitivity and specificity for the diagnosis of follicular carcinoma.

57. d Lymph node involvement.

58. a Total thyroidectomy.

59. b Solitary thyroid nodule.

60. b Thyroglobulin.

61. d Hürthle cell tumour.

62. b 80% of the cases are familial.

63. d b and c.

64. b Surgical resection is possible in most of the patients.

65. b Sub-acute thyroiditis.

66. c Papillary carcinoma.

67. c Hashimoto's thyroiditis.

68. a External branch of superficial laryngeal nerve.

69. c Ligation and division of the superior thyroid vessels.

70. c Zona recticularis.

71. b Iatrogenic.

72. b Hyponatraemia.

73. d Oedema.

74. a Hypoglycaemia.

75. a Ectopic secretion of ACTH.

76. d High-dose dexamethasone suppression test.

77. a Hypersecretion of ACTH.

78. b Most of them are non-functional.

79. a Mitotane.

80. b Benign.

81. d All of the above.

82. b Most of them are familial.

83. a Hypertension.

84. b α-blockers followed by β-blockers.

85. a Metaiodobenzylguanidine (MIBG) scan.

86. b α-blockers followed by caesarean section with or without synchronous adrenalectomy.

87. a Adrenal adenoma.

88. a Zona glomerulosa.

89. d Conn's syndrome.

90. a Spironolactone.

91. a Hypokalaemia.

92. c Addisonian crisis.

93. d Parathyroid adenomas.

94. d b and c.

95. a Prolactinomas.

96. d Phaeochromocytomas.

97. a Tumour size >3 cm.

98. d Dopamine agonists.

99. d Normal gastrin levels exclude the diagnosis of gastrinoma.

100. c Pituitary adenoma.

101. d All of the above.

102. c Benign and solitary.

103. a Hyperglycaemia.

104. b Small bowel.

105. a All patients with jejunoileal carcinoids present with carcinoid syndrome.

106. b Right hemicolectomy.

107. a Local excision.

108. b Octreotide scan is very useful in the diagnosis of rectal carcinoids.

109. d Metaiodobenzylguanidine (MIBG) scan.

110. b Norepinephrine.

111. c Medulloblastoma.

112. a Hypernatraemia, hypokalaemia, metabolic alkalosis.

113. d All of the above.

114. a Adrenal adenoma.

115. c Hypertension.

116. c Tryptophan.

117. b 4:1.

2
Colorectal surgery

Questions

✓ 1. The life-time risk of colorectal cancer in the UK population is:
   a 5%.
   b 10%.
   c 15%.
   d 25%.

2. Which one of the following statements is true regarding the risk of colorectal cancer in a 35-year-old male with no past medical history of colorectal cancer and one first-degree relative with colon cancer diagnosed at 50 years of age?
   a He is at high risk of developing colorectal cancer.
   b He is at moderate risk of developing colorectal cancer.
   c He is at low risk of developing colorectal cancer.
   d None of the above.

3. The risk of colorectal cancer is high in all of the following groups of patients, except:
   a One first-degree relative with bowel cancer diagnosed at 50 years of age.
   b Family history of familial adenomatous polyposis (FAP).
   c Family history of Lynch syndrome.
   d One first-degree relative with bowel cancer diagnosed at the age of 45 years.

✓ 4. The most common inherited large bowel cancer syndrome is:
   a Familial adenomatous polyposis (FAP).
   b Peutz-Jeghers syndrome.
   c Gardner's syndrome.
   d Lynch syndrome.

5. The characteristic features of Lynch syndrome include all of the following, except:
   a Average age at the time of diagnosis is 45 years.
   b Tumours are usually associated with colonic polyps.
   c Tumours have predilection for proximal colon.
   d Tumours tend to be poorly differentiated.

6. Which of the following cancers is not associated with Lynch syndrome?
   a Colonic carcinoma.
   b Medullary carcinoma of thyroid.
   c Endometrial carcinoma.
   d Gastric carcinoma.

7. Which of the following cancer syndromes is not associated with colonic polyps?
   a Familial adenomatous polyposis (FAP).
   b Turcot's syndrome.
   c Gardner's syndrome.
   d Lynch syndrome.

8. The genetic defect associated with Lynch syndrome is:
   a Mutation in the p53 tumour suppressor gene.
   b Germline mutations of mismatch repair genes.
   c Mutation in the cyclin D1 gene.
   d Mutation in the gene for β-cadherin.

9. A patient with a family history of Lynch syndrome and positive genetic testing for microsatellite instability should be offered surveillance colonoscopy:
   a Every 1–2 years from 5 years earlier than the age of the youngest affected relative.
   b Every 3–5 years from the age of 25 years.
   c Every 6 months from the age of 25 years.
   d Every 12 months from the age of 25 years.

10. The investigation that is not recommended as a part of surveillance for extracolonic manifestations of Lynch syndrome is:
    a Mammography every 2 years.
    b Upper gastrointestinal endoscopy every 5 years.
    c Annual urine analysis and cytology.
    d Annual liver function tests, carcinoembryonic antigen and CA 19.9.

11. The treatment of choice in a 45-year-old male patient with caecal and rectal cancer and positive germline mutations for mismatch repair gene is:
    a Right hemicolectomy and anterior resection.
    b Subtotal colectomy.
    c Proctocolectomy with or without ileoanal pouch.
    d Right hemicolectomy and transanal endoscopic microsurgery.

12. The risk of colorectal cancer in patients with familial adenomatous polyposis (FAP) is:
    a 100%.
    b 50%.
    c 75%.
    d 90%.

13. Familial adenomatous polyposis (FAP) is characterised by:
    a The presence of more than one hundred adenomatous polyps.
    b Duodenal polyps.
    c Multiple extra-intestinal manifestations.
    d All of the above.

14. Familial adenomatous polyposis (FAP) is due to:
    a Mutation of p53 gene.
    b Mutation of K-ras gene.
    c Mutation of adenomatous polyposis coli (APC) gene.
    d Mutation of mismatch repair gene.

15. The most appropriate time for colonic surveillance in patients with a family history of familial adenomatous polyposis (FAP) is:
    a 6-monthly flexible sigmoidoscopy starting at the age of 25 years.
    b Annual colonoscopy starting at the age of 20 years.
    c Surveillance should only be offered to patients with a history of rectal bleeding or change of bowel habits or anaemia.
    d 6-monthly flexible sigmoidoscopy starting at the age of 13–15 years.

16. The risk of duodenal malignancy in duodenal adenoma associated with familial adenomatous polyposis (FAP) is:
    a 100%.
    b 5%.
    c 20–30%.
    d 1–2%.

17. The most common site of ischaemic colitis is:
    a Splenic flexure.
    b Transverse colon.
    c Hepatic flexure.
    d Ileocaecal junction.

18. The recommended time interval for endoscopic follow-up of a patient with Spigelman stage 3 duodenal polyposis is:
    a Every 5 years.
    b Every 3 years.
    c Every year.
    d Every 6 months.

19. The difference between MYH-associated colon cancers and familial adenomatous polyposis (FAP) syndrome-associated colon cancers is:
    a It occurs on the right side.
    b It is common at a younger age.
    c It is common in males.
    d None of the above.

20. The type of polyps associated with Peutz-Jeghers syndrome are:
    a Adenomatous polyps.
    b Pseudopolyps.
    c Hamartomatous polyps.
    d Hyperplastic polyps.

21. Which of the following polyps has a high risk of malignant transformation?
    a Flat adenomatous polyps.
    b Polypoid adenomas.
    c Pseudopolyps.
    d Hamartomatous polyps.

22. According to BSG (British Society of Gastroenterology) guidelines, patients with more than five small adenomas should be offered repeat colonoscopy at:
    a 1 year.
    b 3 years.
    c 5 years.
    d 6 months.

23. The strongest layer of small bowel is:
    a Serosa.
    b Submucosa.
    c Mucosa.
    d Muscularis mucosa.

24. The most common site of colorectal cancer is:
    a Right colon.
    b Transverse colon.
    c Left colon.
    d Rectum.

25. Which of the following statements is incorrect regarding mechanical bowel preparation?
    a It prevents anastomotic leak.
    b It can cause severe dehydration in elderly people.
    c It is contraindicated in patients with obstruction.
    d It does not prevent wound infection.

26. Most gastrointestinal anastomotic leaks are due to:
    a Not administrating antibiotics at induction of anaesthesia.
    b Diabetes.
    c Anaemia.
    d Poor anastomotic technique.

27. Colonic bleeding secondary to angiodysplasia is characterised by all of the following features, except:
    a It is associated with intermittent fresh red rectal bleeding.
    b It can be associated with underlying aortic stenosis.
    c It can be associated with iron deficiency anaemia.
    d Sigmoid colon is the most commonly affected site.

28. The minimum number of lymph nodes required for the evaluation of lymph node staging in patients with colorectal cancer is:
a 12.
b 6.
c 3.
d 24.

29. Prophylactic antibiotics should be given:
a Immediately after induction.
b At the time of bowel anastomosis.
c An hour before induction.
d Immediately after skin incision.

30. The colorectal cancer that is associated with a high local recurrence rate and poor survival is:
a Caecal cancer.
b Sigmoid cancer.
c Rectal cancer.
d Splenic flexure cancer.

31. In a 45-year-old male recently diagnosed with caecal cancer, staging computed tomography showed a large caecal tumour involving the right ureter and lower pole of right kidney. The best treatment option would be:
a Chemoradiotherapy followed by surgery.
b Right hemicolectomy and right nephrectomy.
c Ileocolic bypass.
d Palliative chemotherapy.

32. A 70-year-old female patient underwent anterior resection with primary anastomosis 5 days ago. She is suspected to have anastomotic leak on the sixth post-operative day. The most appropriate investigation to confirm an anastomotic leak is:
a Barium enema.
b CT of the abdomen.
c Water-soluble contrast enema.
d CT of the abdomen with a contrast enema.

33. The chance of lymph node involvement is high in which one of the following types of colorectal cancer:
    a Moderately-differentiated colorectal cancer confined to the bowel wall.
    b Poorly-differentiated colorectal cancer penetrating the full thickness of the bowel wall.
    c Well-differentiated colorectal cancer penetrating the full thickness of the bowel wall.
    d Poorly-differentiated colorectal cancer confined to the bowel wall.

34. The incidence of synchronous lesions in patients with rectal cancer is:
    a 10%.
    b 15%.
    c 3%.
    d 1%.

35. The investigation of choice for loco-regional assessment of rectal cancer is:
    a Magnetic resonance imaging (MRI).
    b CT scan.
    c Endorectal ultrasound.
    d Positron emission tomography (PET)-CT.

36. Which of the following group of patients is at high risk of developing side-effects due to 5-fluorouracil (FU)?
    a Patients with deficiency of thymidylate synthase.
    b Patients with dihydropyrimidine dehydrogenase deficiency.
    c Patients with deficiency of topoisomerase I.
    d Patients with deficiency of thymidine phosphate.

37. Which of the following features is associated with worst prognosis in stage-II colon cancer?
    a Perforation.
    b Obstruction.
    c Poorly-differentiated tumours.
    d Involvement of peritoneum.
    e All of the above.

38. The rationale behind the use of radiotherapy in patients with rectal cancer include all except:
   a To reduce the local recurrence.
   b To reduce the distant spread.
   c To downstage the tumour to achieve sphincter preserving surgery.
   d To downstage the tumour to allow successful resection.

39. The advantage of pre-operative radiotherapy compared to post-operative radiotherapy in rectal carcinoma is:
   a Pelvic anatomy is undisturbed.
   b Less small bowel in radiation field.
   c Reduced gastrointestinal toxicity.
   d All of the above.
   e None of the above.

40. All of the following are long-term complications associated with a short course of pre-operative radiotherapy, except:
   a Permanent sterility.
   b Erectile dysfunction.
   c Impaired bowel function.
   d Pelvic fracture.

41. Which part of the colon is most commonly affected by ulcerative colitis?
   a Rectum.
   b Sigmoid colon.
   c Transverse colon.
   d Right colon.

42. The most common extra-intestinal manifestation of ulcerative colitis is:
   a Primary sclerosing colitis.
   b Erythema nodosum.
   c Uveitis.
   d Arthropathy.

43. Primary sclerosing cholangitis associated with inflammatory bowel syndrome is characterised by all of the following features, except:
    a Primary sclerosing cholangitis is more commonly associated with ulcerative colitis than Crohn's disease.
    b Cholangiocarcinoma is common in patients with ulcerative colitis.
    c The risk of cholangiocarcinoma is similar before and after proctocolectomy in patients with ulcerative colitis.
    d None of the above.

44. The features which differentiate ulcerative colitis and Crohn's disease include all of the following, except:
    a Rectal sparing is common in ulcerative colitis.
    b Anal disease is common in ulcerative colitis.
    c Intestinal fistulisation is uncommon in ulcerative colitis.
    d Full thickness bowel wall involvement is not a feature of ulcerative colitis.

45. Ulcerative colitis is characterised by:
    a Involvement of the mucosa and submucosa.
    b Rectal sparing.
    c Stricture formation.
    d Cryptic abscess formation.
    e a and d.

46. Infliximab is a synthetic:
    a Anti-TNF-α monoclonal antibody.
    b IL-2 receptor inhibitor.
    c Anti-TNF-β monoclonal antibody.
    d IL-6 receptor inhibitor.

47. Indications for surgery in patients with acute colitis include:
    a Failed medical treatment.
    b Presence of megacolon.
    c Bloody diarrhoea >10 times in 24 hours.
    d All of the above.

48. The operation of choice in a patient with acute colitis is:
    a Sub-total colectomy with ileostomy.
    b Proctocolectomy with an ileoanal pouch.
    c Subtotal colectomy with ileoanal anastomosis.
    d Proctocolectomy with end ileostomy.

49. The indications for emergency surgery in patients with colitis include:
    a Poor compliance.
    b Recurrent acute exacerbations.
    c Growth retardation.
    d Toxic megacolon.

50. Extra-intestinal manifestations of ulcerative colitis that respond to colonic resection are:
    a Polyarthropathy.
    b Erythema nodosum.
    c Pyoderma gangrenosum.
    d All of the above.

51. The contraindications for a restorative proctocolectomy with ileo-anal pouch is:
    a Ulcerative colitis.
    b Crohn's colitis.
    c Familial adenomatous polyposis.
    d Indeterminate colitis.

52. The incidence of colorectal cancer in patients with colitis of less than 10 years duration is:
    a Nil.
    b 10–15%.
    c 20%.
    d 50%.

53. Crohn's disease commonly affects the:
    a Small bowel.
    b Colon.
    c Perianal area.
    d Duodenum.

54. The active component of salazopyrin is:
a   Aspirin.
b   Sulphonamide.
c   5-aminosalicylic acid (ASA).
d   Salazopyrin.

55. The earliest macroscopic lesions found in patients with Crohn's disease are:
a   Apthous ulcers.
b   Inflammatory polyps.
c   Stricture formation.
d   Loss of mucosal vascular pattern.

56. All of the following are extra-intestinal manifestations related to Crohn's disease activity, except:
a   Pyoderma gangrenosum.
b   Erythema nodosum.
c   Gallstones.
d   Acute arthropathy.

57. The most frequent indication for surgery in patients with Crohn's disease is:
a   Perianal disease.
b   Intestinal fistula.
c   Small bowel obstruction.
d   Crohn's colitis.

58. Crohn's disease is a contraindication for an ileoanal pouch because of the:
a   High risk of cancer in the pouch.
b   High risk of pouchitis.
c   Risk of recurrence of Crohn's disease in the small bowel/perianal area.
d   Future risk of small bowel resection following recurrence.

59. A 25-year-old female underwent incision drainage for a perianal abscess 6 months ago. She re-presents with persistent purulent discharge from the incisional drainage site in the last 2 weeks. The next step in the management of this patient is:
   a Examination under anaesthesia.
   b CT scan of pelvis.
   c Magnetic resonance imaging (MRI) of pelvis.
   d Small bowel enema followed by examination under anaesthesia.

60. A fistula is a:
   a Communication between two epithelial lined surfaces.
   b Communication between epithelial and non-epithelial lined surfaces.
   c Communication between two non-epithelial lined surfaces.
   d Blind-ending tract.

61. The presence of skin organisms in the pus obtained from a perianal abscess indicates that:
   a The risk of fistula formation is extremely low.
   b The risk of fistula formation is high.
   c There is an underlying inflammatory bowel disease.
   d The risk of recurrence of a perianal abscess is high.

62. A 25-year-old female patient presents with painful perianal swelling present for the last 3 days. On examination under anaesthesia, she is found to have a perianal abscess and a low fistula in ano. The treatment of choice is:
   a Incision and drainage of abscess.
   b Incision, drainage and fistulotomy.
   c Incision, drainage and seton insertion.
   d Incision and drainage followed by magnetic resonance imaging (MRI).

63. According to Goodsall's rule the site of the internal opening of a fistula in ano can be predicted by:
   a The position of the external opening.
   b The distance of the external opening from the anal verge.
   c The absence of induration.
   d None of the above.

64. Exceptions to Goodsall's rule include all of the following, except:
    a Posteriorly located external opening of fistula.
    b Anteriorly located external opening of fistula >3 cm from anal verge.
    c The presence of underlying Crohn's disease.
    d The presence of underlying malignancy.

65. The common type of perianal fistula is:
    a Intersphincteric.
    b Transsphincteric.
    c Suprasphincteric.
    d Extrasphincteric.

66. Seton insertion should be considered in patients with:
    a Fistula in ano with multiple external openings.
    b Low fistula in ano.
    c High fistula in ano.
    d b and c.
    e a and c.

67. A seton helps in the management of fistula in ano by:
    a Allowing free drainage of pus.
    b Allowing cutting and healing of the external sphincter.
    c Acting as a marker for fistula tract.
    d All of the above.

68. The loose seton can be used:
    a To preserve the entire external sphincter.
    b To preserve part of the voluntary muscle.
    c As part of staged fistulotomy.
    d All of the above.

69. The contraindication for the use of anal advancement flap for the treatment of fistula in ano is:
    a Presence of acute sepsis.
    b Internal opening <2.5 cm from dentate line.
    c Previous incision and drainage.
    d Diabetes.

70. Anal cushions are:
    a Normal functional structures contributing to anal continence.
    b Abnormal arteriovenous complexes.
    c Abnormal structures found in the anal canal.
    d a and c.

71. The treatment of choice for grade II haemorrhoids is:
    a Rubber band ligation.
    b Open haemorrhoidectomy.
    c Electro-coagulation.
    d Stool softener.

72. Which of the following is a common site of polyps in patients with
    Peutz-Jeghers syndrome?
    a Large bowel.
    b Small bowel.
    c Rectum.
    d Stomach.

73. Colonic pseudo-obstruction can be temporarily relieved by the
    administration of:
    a Neostigmine.
    b Atropine.
    c Metoclopramide.
    d Cisapride.

74. Stapled haemorrhoidectomy is associated with all of the following,
    except:
    a It corrects the underlying pathophysiology.
    b It alleviates symptoms.
    c It is associated with an increased recurrence of symptoms in the
      long term.
    d It is not useful in prolapsed haemorrhoids.

75. Secondary bleeding following haemorrhoidectomy is due to:
    a Infection.
    b Slipping of ligature.
    c Recurrence of haemorrhoid.
    d Straining.

76. The most common early complication following haemorrhoidectomy in male patients is:
   a Urinary retention.
   b Reactionary haemorrhage.
   c Faecal incontinence.
   d Anal stricture.

77. All of the following features suggest chronicity of an anal fissure,
   except:
   a Presence of anal skin tag.
   b Presence of fibroepithelial polyp.
   c Presence of symptoms >6 weeks.
   d a and b.

78. The most common site of an anterior anal fissure is at:
   a 9 o'clock.
   b 6 o'clock.
   c 3 o'clock.
   d 12 o'clock.

79. The most common site of an anal fissure in post-partum females is:
   a 6 o'clock.
   b 9 o'clock.
   c 3 o'clock.
   d 12 o'clock.

80. The treatment of choice for anal fissure is:
   a Surgery.
   b Botulinum toxin.
   c Anal dilatation.
   d GTN ointment.

81. The most effective treatment for anal fissure is:
   a Lateral sphincterotomy.
   b Botulinum toxin.
   c GTN ointment.
   d Diltiazem ointment.

82. The percentage GTN ointment used in the treatment of anal fissure is:
    a 0.2%.
    b 0.5%.
    c 1%.
    d 1.2%.

83. The common side-effect associated with GTN ointment is:
    a Headache.
    b Hypotension.
    c Cough.
    d Sweating.

84. Intestinal failure is more likely to occur in a patient with small bowel of less than:
    a 100 cm in the presence of ileostomy.
    b 100 cm in the presence of colon.
    c 150 cm in the presence of ileostomy.
    d 150 cm in the presence of colon.

85. The rationale for the administration of sodium along with glucose in patients with severe dehydration due to intestinal failure is:
    a Sodium absorption is linked to the absorption of glucose.
    b The majority of these patients are hypoglycaemic.
    c Glucose prevents the excretion of sodium.
    d Sodium helps the metabolism of glucose.

86. Sodium absorption normally occurs in the:
    a Ileum and colon.
    b Duodenum.
    c Proximal jejunum.
    d Stomach.

87. Magnesium is usually absorbed in the:
    a Duodenum.
    b Stomach.
    c Distal jejunum and ileum.
    d Colon.

88. The most common source of vitamin K is:
    a Intestinal bacteria.
    b Meat products.
    c Dairy products.
    d Vegetables.

89. All of the following are constituents of St Mark's solution, except:
    a Glucose.
    b Potassium chloride.
    c Sodium chloride.
    d Sodium bicarbonate.

90. Complications associated with total parenteral nutrition include:
    a Gallstones.
    b Hyperglycaemia.
    c Hyperkalaemia.
    d All of the above.

91. Most anal cancers originate from the:
    a Anal glands.
    b Anal ducts.
    c Squamous epithelial lining.
    d Columnar epithelial lining.

92. The most common type of anal tumour is:
    a Squamous cell carcinoma.
    b Lymphoma.
    c Malignant melanoma.
    d Adenocarcinoma.

93. The human papilloma virus strains associated with anal carcinoma are:
    a Types 16, 18, 31 and 33.
    b Types 6 and 11.
    c Types 4 and 8.
    d Types 36 and 38.

94. Anogenital intra-epithelial neoplasia is graded from I to III according to the:
    a Degree of differentiation.
    b Number of thirds of epithelial cell depth that are dysplastic.
    c Number of mitotic figures.
    d Degree of lymphovascular invasion.

95. Basaloid tumours of the anal canal arise from the:
a Anal verge.
b Transitional zone of the anal canal.
c Anal canal area covered by rectal mucosa.
d None of the above.

96. The treatment of choice for anal carcinoma is:
a Chemoradiotherapy.
b Chemotherapy.
c Radiotherapy.
d Radical excision.

97. Which one of the following anal tumours has the worst prognosis?
a Squamous cell carcinoma.
b Adenocarcinoma.
c Lymphoma.
d Melanoma.

98. Which of the following is not an indication for the use of pre-operative chemoradiotherapy in patients with rectal cancer?
a Tumour shrinkage.
b Reduced local recurrence.
c Treatment of micro-metastasis.
d Reduced anastomotic leak rate.

99. The most likely diagnosis in a young male patient presenting with acute abdominal pain, blood and mucus in his stool and with a palpable mass per abdomen is due to:
a Meckel's diverticulum.
b Volvulus.
c Intussusception.
d Hypertrophic pyloric stenosis.

100. Faecal continence is normally maintained by all of the following, except:
a Anorectal angulation.
b Rectal innervations.
c Internal anal sphincter.
d Haustral valves.

101. Meckel's diverticulum is a remnant of:
    a Stenson's duct.
    b Wolffian duct.
    c Mullerian duct.
    d Vitello-intestinal duct.

102. The best method of diagnosis of ectopic gastric mucosa of Meckel's diverticulum is:
    a Fluoroscopy.
    b Occult blood test in the stool.
    c Ultrasound of the abdomen.
    d Radionuclide scan.

103. The most common neoplasm of the appendix is:
    a Lymphoma.
    b Adenocarcinoma.
    c Leiomyosarcoma.
    d Argentaffinoma.

104. The nerve most commonly damaged during McBurney's incision is the:
    a Subcostal nerve.
    b Iliohypogastric nerve.
    c 11th thoracic nerve.
    d 10th thoracic nerve.

105. The most common position of the appendix is:
    a Retrocaecal.
    b Pre-ileal.
    c Paracaecal.
    d Post-ileal.

106. The most common tumour of the small intestine is:
    a Leiomyoma.
    b Lymphoma.
    c Adenocarcinoma.
    d Haemangioma.

107. Pseudomyxoma peritonei is seen with which of the following
conditions?
a Thecoma ovary.
b Mucin secreting ovarian carcinoma.
c Carcinoid appendix.
d Mesothelioma.

Answers: Colorectal surgery

1. a 5%.

2. c He is at low risk of developing colorectal cancer.

3. a One first-degree relative with bowel cancer diagnosed at 50 years of age.

4. d Lynch syndrome.

5. b Tumours are usually associated with colonic polyps.

6. b Medullary carcinoma of thyroid.

7. d Lynch syndrome.

8. b Germline mutations of mismatch repair genes.

9. a Every 1–2 years from 5 years earlier than the age of the youngest affected relative.

10. a Mammography every 2 years.

11. c Proctocolectomy with or without ileoanal pouch.

12. a 100%.

13. d All of the above.

14. c Mutation of adenomatous polyposis coli (APC) gene.

15. d 6-monthly flexible sigmoidoscopy starting at the age of 13–15 years.

16. b 5%.

17. a Splenic flexure.

18. c Every year.

19. a It occurs on the right side.

20. c Hamartomatous polyps.

21. a Flat adenomatous polyps.

22. a 1 year.

23. b Submucosa.

24. c Left colon.

25. a It prevents anastomotic leak.

26. d Poor anastomotic technique.

27. d Sigmoid colon is the most commonly affected site.

28. a 12.

29. a Immediately after induction.

30. c Rectal cancer.

31. b Right hemicolectomy and right nephrectomy.

32. d CT of the abdomen with a contrast enema.

33. b Poorly-differentiated colorectal cancer penetrating the full thickness of the bowel wall.

34. c 3%.

35. a Magnetic resonance imaging (MRI).

36. b Patients with dihydropyrimidine dehydrogenase deficiency.

37. e All of the above.

38. b To reduce the distant spread.

39. d All of the above.

40. d Pelvic fracture.

41. a Rectum.

42. d Arthropathy.

43. b Cholangiocarcinoma is common in patients with ulcerative colitis.

44. b Anal disease is common in ulcerative colitis.

45. e a and d.

46. a Anti-TNF-α monoclonal antibody.

47. d All of the above.

48. c Subtotal colectomy with ileoanal anastomosis.

49. d Toxic megacolon.

50. d All of the above.

51. b Crohn's colitis.

52. a Nil.

53. c Perianal area.

54. c 5-aminosalicylic acid (ASA).

55. a Apthous ulcers.

56. c Gallstones.

57. c Small bowel obstruction.

58. c Risk of recurrence of Crohn's disease in the small bowel/perianal area.

59. a Examination under anaesthesia.

60. a Communication between two epithelial lined surfaces.

61. a The risk of fistula formation is extremely low.

62. b Incision, drainage and fistulotomy.

63. a The position of the external opening.

64. a Posteriorly located external opening of fistula.

65. a Intersphincteric.

66. e a and c.

67. d All of the above.

68. d All of the above.

69. a Presence of acute sepsis.

70. a Normal functional structures contributing to anal continence.

71. a Rubber band ligation.

72. b Small bowel.

73. a Neostigmine.

74. d It is not useful in prolapsed haemorrhoids.

75. a Infection.

76. a Urinary retention.

77. **d** a and b.

78. **b** 6 o'clock.

79. **d** 12 o'clock.

80. **d** GTN ointment.

81. **a** Lateral sphincterotomy.

82. **a** 0.2%.

83. **a** Headache.

84. **a** 100 cm in the presence of ileostomy.

85. **a** Sodium absorption is linked to the absorption of glucose.

86. **a** Ileum and colon.

87. **c** Distal jejunum and ileum.

88. **a** Intestinal bacteria.

89. **b** Potassium chloride.

90. **d** All of the above.

91. **c** Squamous epithelial lining.

92. **a** Squamous cell carcinoma.

93. **a** Types 16, 18, 31 and 33.

94. **b** Number of thirds of epithelial cell depth that are dysplastic.

95. **b** Transitional zone of the anal canal.

96. **a** Chemoradiotherapy.

97. **d** Melanoma.

98. d Reduced anastomotic leak rate.

99. c Intussusception.

100. d Haustral valves.

101. d Vitello-intestinal duct.

102. d Radionuclide scan.

103. d Argentaffinoma.

104. b Iliohypogastric nerve.

105. a Retrocaecal.

106. a Leiomyoma.

107. b Mucin secreting ovarian carcinoma.

3

Oesophagogastric surgery

Questions

1. All of the following are predisposing factors for oesophageal cancer, except:
   a Achalasia.
   b Tylosis.
   c Corrosive stricture.
   d *Helicobacter pylori* infection.

2. The most common type of oesophageal malignancy associated with Barrett's oesophagus is:
   a Adenocarcinoma.
   b Squamous cell carcinoma.
   c Adenosquamous cell carcinoma.
   d Lymphoma.

3. The most common site of the oesophageal carcinoma is:
   a Upper third thoracic oesophagus.
   b Middle third thoracic oesophagus.
   c Lower third thoracic oesophagus.
   d Cervical oesophagus.

4. The most common type of gastric polyps are:
   a Hyperplastic polyps.
   b Fundic polyps.
   c Neoplastic polyps.
   d Inflammatory polyps.

5. The gastric polyp that has no risk of malignant transformation is:
    a Adenomatous polyp.
    b Hyperplastic polyp.
    c Fundic gland polyp.
    d Polyp associated with familial adenomatous polyp.

6. Early gastric cancer is defined as:
    a Carcinoma limited to mucosa or submucosa with lymph node involvement.
    b Carcinoma limited to mucosa or submucosa without lymph node involvement.
    c Carcinoma limited to mucosa or submucosa irrespective of lymph node involvement.
    d Full thickness involvement of the stomach without lymph node involvement.

7. The most common type of early gastric cancer is:
    a Ulcerating type (type III and IIc).
    b Exophytic type.
    c Flat type.
    d Elevated type (type IIa).

8. Which one of the following statements is incorrect with regard to early gastric cancer?
    a They are predominantly found in the fundus of the stomach.
    b 5-year survival is over 90%.
    c Intramucosal early gastric cancers are rarely associated with lymph node involvement.
    d Ulcerative type (type III and IIc) is the most common type.

9. Familial gastric cancer is associated with germline mutations of which of the following genes:
    a p53.
    b APC.
    c DCC.
    d E-cadherin.

10. The most common site of gastrointestinal stromal tumours is:
    a Stomach.
    b Small bowel.
    c Large bowel.
    d Rectum.

11. The most common site of extranodal lymphoma is:
    a Oesophagus.
    b Stomach.
    c Duodenum.
    d Ileum.

12. The treatment of choice for stage I mucosa-associated lymphatic tissue lymphoma (MALToma) is:
    a *Helicobacter pylori* eradication.
    b Sub-total gastrectomy.
    c Total gastrectomy.
    d Systemic chemotherapy and radiotherapy.

13. The incidence of carcinoma is high in gastric polyps of size more than:
    a 1 cm.
    b 2 cm.
    c 3 cm.
    d 5 cm.

14. Which of the following conditions is associated with an increased risk of cervical oesophageal cancer?
    a Plummer-Vinson syndrome.
    b Achalasia cardia.
    c Barrett's oesophagus.
    d Gastro-oesophageal reflux.

15. The investigation associated with high sensitivity and specificity in the loco-regional staging of oesophageal cancer is:
    a Endoscopic ultrasound (EUS).
    b Computed tomography (CT).
    c Magnetic resonance imaging (MRI).
    d Positron emission tomography (PET)-CT.

16. The commonly used in vitro dye stains for the detection of early oesophageal cancer are:
    a 1–2% Lugol's iodine.
    b 2% toluidine blue.
    c 1–2% methylene blue.
    d All of the above.

17. *Helicobacter pylori* is not associated with:
    a Mucosa-associated lymphatic tissue lymphoma (MALToma).
    b Gastric cancer.
    c Gastric leiomyoma.
    d Gastric ulcer.

18. Positron emission tomography (PET) differs from computed tomography (CT) and magnetic resonance imaging (MRI) in all of the following aspects, except:
    a It gives anatomical details of the tumour.
    b It measures the biological and physiological function of the tumour tissue.
    c It can predict the response to chemotherapy.
    d It is based on the high metabolic activity of the malignant cells.

19. The following investigation has better specificity and sensitivity in detecting nodal and distant metastasis of oesophageal cancer:
    a Magnetic resonance imaging (MRI).
    b Endoscopic ultrasound (EUS).
    c CT scan.
    d Positron emission tomography (PET) scan.
    e PET-CT.

20. The most accurate staging modality for T and local N staging of oesophageal cancer is:
    a Positron emission tomography (PET)-CT.
    b Endoscopic ultrasound (EUS).
    c CT scan.
    d Magnetic resonance imaging (MRI).

21. The presence of which of the following features is highly indicative of lymph nodal involvement on endoscopic ultrasound:
    a Rounded, sharply demarcated, homogenous, hypoechoic.
    b Elongated, heterogenous, hyperechoic with indistinct borders.
    c Lymph nodes of more than 8 mm in size.
    d Rounded, heterogenous with distinct borders.

22. The most common site of a benign (peptic) gastric ulcer is the:
    a Upper third of the lesser curvature.
    b Greater curvature.
    c Pyloric antrum.
    d Lesser curvature near incisura angularis.

23. Staging laparoscopy is indicated in patients with gastric cancer because:
    a It can detect less than 1 cm liver metastasis.
    b It is more accurate in detecting small peritoneal metastasis.
    c It has the advantage of cytological assessment of tumour spread.
    d All of the above.

24. A 55-year-old male patient with type II diabetes, hypertension and asthma well controlled on medication was recently diagnosed with lower oesophageal cancer. His American Society of Anesthesiologists (ASA) grade would be:
    a ASA-I.
    b ASA-II.
    c ASA-III.
    d ASA-IV.

25. Which of the following statements is incorrect with regard to metabolic equivalents (MET levels)?
    a MET levels are measures of aerobic demand for common daily activity and past-time.
    b One MET level is equivalent to 3.5 mL/kg/min of O_2 uptake in a 70 kg, 40-year-old male at rest.
    c Peri-operative cardiac and long-term risk is increased in patients unable to meet a 4-MET demand during normal activity.
    d The functional capacity is considered excellent if METs are less than seven.

26. The clinical predictors of increased peri-operative cardiovascular risk in patients undergoing major oesophageal resectional surgery are:
    a Myocardial infarction within 6 months prior to surgery.
    b Unstable angina.
    c Diabetes mellitus.
    d a and b.

27. All of the following are clinical predictors of significant peri-operative cardiovascular risk, except:
   a Patients who had recent coronary artery bypass graft (CABG) surgery with good residual ventricular function.
   b Severe aortic valvular disease.
   c Decompensated congestive heart failure.
   d High-grade arterioventricular block.

28. The beneficial effects of smoking cessation in reducing post-operative morbidity are only seen in patients:
   a Who stop smoking 8 weeks before surgery.
   b Who stop smoking within a month prior to surgery.
   c Who stop smoking 2 weeks prior to surgery.
   d Who stop smoking within 48 hours before surgery.

29. Which of the following statements is incorrect with regard to lymphatic spread in patients with early oesophageal cancer?
   a Lymph node metastasis is rare in tumours limited to mucosa.
   b The prevalence of lymph node metastasis increases to 25% by invasion into the submucosa.
   c High-grade dysplasia is not associated with lymphatic spread.
   d 5–10% of patients with pT1a have lymph node metastasis.

30. The advantages of the transhiatal approach compared to the transthoracic approach include all, except:
   a Associated with lower risk of respiratory complications.
   b Associated with higher risk of anastomotic leak.
   c Radical thoracic lymph node clearance is better.
   d It is the preferred approach in patients with early oesophageal cancer.

31. The best oesophageal conduit is:
   a Stomach.
   b Jejunum.
   c Colon.
   d Free jejunal graft.

32. The most common complication following oesophagectomy is:
   a Anastomotic leak.
   b Chyle leak.
   c Pneumonia.
   d Anastomotic stricture.

33. The most effective and preferred treatment for cervical oesophageal cancer is:
    a Total pharyngolaryngectomy.
    b Total oesophagectomy with anastomosis in neck.
    c Chemoradiotherapy.
    d Chemotherapy followed by surgery.

34. Which of the following statements is incorrect with regard to familial gastric cancer due to E-cadherin gene mutation?
    a Diffuse type is more common.
    b It is an autosomal recessive disorder.
    c It is associated with poor prognosis.
    d Mutant gene carriers may also develop breast or colorectal carcinoma.

35. Early gastric cancer with the following features is not suitable for endoscopic mucosal resection (EMR):
    a Elevated or flat lesions less than 2 cm.
    b Depressed lesion less than 1 cm without ulceration.
    c Poorly-differentiated tumour.
    d Lesion confined to mucosa.

36. The thoracic duct enters the posterior mediastinum through the following opening in the diaphragm:
    a Aorta.
    b Oesophagus.
    c Inferior vena cava.
    d It has a separate opening in the diaphragm.

37. The oesophageal opening in the diaphragm corresponds to:
    a T10.
    b T12.
    c T8.
    d L1.

38. The strongest layer in the oesophagus is the:
    a Mucosa.
    b Submucosa.
    c Muscularis propria.
    d Serosa.

39. Which of the following is an incorrect statement regarding the anatomy of the thoracic oesophagus?
   a The azygous vein passes posterior to the oesophagus before joining the superior vena cava.
   b The thoracic duct is related to the posterolateral aspect of the oesophagus.
   c It has no serosal covering.
   d The lower third of the oesophagus is anteriorly related to the pericardium.

40. The preferred route of reconstruction following primary surgical excision of oesophageal cancer is:
   a Pre-sternal.
   b Retro-sternal.
   c Through posterior mediastinum.
   d All of the above.

41. The posterior mediastinal route is the preferred route of oesophageal reconstruction following oesophageal resection because:
   a Anastomotic leak rate is low compared to the retro-sternal route.
   b The retro-sternal route may result in unpleasant sensation during swallowing.
   c It provides the shortest distance between the abdomen and apex of thorax.
   d b and c.

42. The stomach is the most commonly used conduit for reconstruction following oesophagectomy. In the preparation of gastric conduit, the following blood vessels are preserved:
   a Left gastric artery.
   b Right gastric artery.
   c Short gastric vessels.
   d Right gastric artery and gastroepiploic arcade.

43. A 50-year-old male patient with a previous history of gastric resection surgery for ulcer disease is recently diagnosed with T3N0 gastro-oesophageal cancer. The most preferred conduit in this patient following oesophageal resection is:
   a Stomach.
   b Colon.
   c Jejunum.
   d Free jejunal graft.

44. Mesenteric angiography is indicated in all of the following cases, except:
    a In patients undergoing oesophageal resection with a previous history of gastric resection surgery.
    b In patients undergoing primary oesophageal resection.
    c In patients who had failed oesophageal reconstruction following gastric conduit.
    d b and c.

45. Gastric cancer most commonly spreads via:
    a Direct extension.
    b Lymphatics.
    c Peritoneal.
    d Haematogenous.

46. Which of the following statements is incorrect regarding diffuse gastric cancer?
    a It is common in the upper third of the stomach.
    b It is more common in elderly patients.
    c It is associated with poor prognosis.
    d It is the commonest type of cancer linked with genetic disorder.

47. The reason behind increased morbidity, mortality and poor survival following gastric cancer surgery in the West compared to Japan is mainly due to:
    a It is a different disease in the West.
    b A higher proportion of patients in Japan have intestinal type cancer.
    c The incidence of proximal cancer is higher in the West.
    d b and c.

48. Which of the following lymph node stations are rarely involved in the metastasis from distal gastric cancer?
    a Stations 3 and 4.
    b Stations 5 and 6.
    c Stations 7 and 8.
    d Stations 2 and 10.

49. The risk of nodal metastasis to which of the following lymph node stations is low in patients with middle third gastric cancer?
   a   Stations 3 and 4.
   b   Stations 6 and 7.
   c   Stations 8 and 9.
   d   Stations 2 and 10.

50. Proximal third gastric cancer rarely spreads to which of the following lymph node stations?
   a   Station 1.
   b   Station 7.
   c   Station 3.
   d   Station 12.

51. Which of the following lymph node stations are not removed en bloc in patients with distal third gastric cancer?
   a   Stations 5 and 6.
   b   Stations 2 and 10.
   c   Stations 7 and 8.
   d   Stations 3 and 4.

52. Early dumping syndrome is common following:
   a   Partial gastrectomy.
   b   Total gastrectomy.
   c   Subtotal gastrectomy.
   d   Total gastrectomy and jejunal pouch.

53. Early dumping syndrome is due to:
   a   Rapid movement of fluid into the small intestine from extra-cellular fluid.
   b   Hypoglycaemia.
   c   Reflux of alkaline contents into the stomach.
   d   Bacterial overgrowth.

54. Malabsorption of the following vitamins is common after subtotal/total gastrectomy:
   a   Vitamin A, D and B12.
   b   Vitamin E, C and C.
   c   Vitamin A, E and K.
   d   Vitamin K, D and B12.

55. Which of the following statements regarding gastrointestinal stromal tumours (GIST) is incorrect?
   a   Stomach is the commonest site.
   b   They spread through the lymphatics.
   c   Most GISTs are spindle cell tumours.
   d   They most likely originate from interstitial cells of Cajal.

56. The molecular feature that differentiates gastrointestinal stromal tumours (GIST) from other mesenchymal tumours is:
   a   Presence of CD 117.
   b   Presence of CD 4.
   c   Presence of CD 25.
   d   Presence of CD 8.

57. The parameter that is not useful in the assessment of the prognosis of gastrointestinal stromal tumour (GIST) is:
   a   Size of the tumour.
   b   Mitotic index.
   c   Ki-67 proliferative index.
   d   Location of the tumour.

58. A 50-year-old patient with 8 cm of gastrointestinal stromal tumour (GIST) in the small bowel underwent resection and anastomosis. The histology of the tumour shows a mitotic index of more than 10 per 10 high power fields. The risk of recurrence in this patient is:
   a   Very low.
   b   Low.
   c   Intermediate.
   d   High.

59. Which of the following statements regarding gastrointestinal stromal tumour (GIST) is incorrect?
   a   Benign GISTs are more common in the small bowel.
   b   Gastric GISTs have better survival than GIST arising from other sites.
   c   They commonly metastasise to the liver.
   d   Approximately 3% of GISTs are negative for KIT gene mutation.

60. The investigation useful in assessing response to chemotherapy in patients with gastrointestinal stromal cell tumours (GISTs) is:
   a Computed tomography.
   b Magnetic resonance imaging.
   c Positron emission tomography (PET)-CT.
   d Somatostatin receptor scintigraphy.

61. The preferred type of surgical resection in a patient with approximately 4 cm pedunculated gastrointestinal stromal tumour (GIST) arising from the body of the stomach is:
   a Total gastrectomy.
   b Sub-total gastrectomy.
   c Wedge resection of the stomach.
   d Partial gastrectomy with lymphadenectomy.

62. The mechanism of the action of imatinib used in the treatment of gastrointestinal stromal tumour (GIST) is:
   a It blocks the binding of ATP to c-KIT.
   b It inhibits the downward signalling pathway after the activation of c-KIT.
   c It inhibits the transportation of NF1 into the nucleus.
   d It inhibits the proliferation of cells by arresting the cell cycle in G1/S phase.

63. Imatinib is used in all of the following settings in gastrointestinal stromal tumour (GIST), except:
   a Unresectable GIST.
   b Resectable GIST.
   c As an adjuvant therapy following surgical resection.
   d As neoadjuvant therapy.

64. The main reason for the development of resistance to imatinib in the treatment of gastrointestinal stromal tumour (GIST) is:
   a Presence of KIT exon 9 mutation.
   b Presence of PDGFR α.
   c Due to development of antibodies to imatinib.
   d Due to increased efflux of imatinib.

65. Which of the following statements regarding the anatomy of the oesophagus is incorrect?
   a The lower third of the oesophagus is entirely composed of skeletal muscle.
   b The oesophagus receives blood supply from the inferior thyroid artery, descending thoracic aorta and left gastric artery.
   c The oesophagus is lined by non-keratinised squamous epithelium.
   d It passes through the diaphragm at the level of T10.

66. Corkscrew oesophagus is seen in which one of the following conditions?
   a Carcinoma of the oesophagus.
   b Scleroderma.
   c Achalasia cardia.
   d Diffuse oesophageal spasm.

67. The most predominant cause of symptomatic gastro-oesophageal reflux disease (GORD) is:
   a Hiatus hernia.
   b Inappropriate transient lower oesophageal sphincter relaxations.
   c Inability to clear the acid from the oesophagus.
   d Delayed gastric emptying.

68. Which of the following statements regarding the pathophysiology of gastro-oesophageal reflux disease (GORD) is incorrect?
   a Presence of *Helicobacter pylori* infection is associated with increased acid secretion and GORD.
   b The significance of delayed gastric emptying in the pathogenesis of GORD is unclear.
   c Impaired oesophageal acid clearance can be associated with GORD.
   d At present, the exact role of duodeno-gastric reflux in GORD is unclear.

69. The gold standard test in establishing the diagnosis of gastro-oesophageal reflux disease (GORD) is:
   a Oesophageal manometry.
   b 24-hour ambulatory pH monitoring.
   c Upper GI endoscopy.
   d Double contrast barium swallow.

70. The oesophageal pH of less than 4, recorded 5 cm above a mano-metrically defined lower oesophageal sphincter should be present in:
   a <4% of 24-hour period in normal individuals.
   b <25% of 24-hour period in normal individuals.
   c <50% of 24-hour period in normal individuals.
   d <10% of 24-hour period in normal individuals.

71. The most useful parameter for the diagnosis of gastro-oesophageal reflux disease (GORD) in a 24-hour pH study is:
   a Total acid reflux time.
   b Acid reflux time during supine position.
   c Acid reflux time during sleeping.
   d Acid reflux time after meals.

72. Auerbach's plexus is situated:
   a Between the outer longitudinal and inner circular muscle of the oesophagus.
   b In the submucosa of the oesophagus.
   c In the muscularis mucosa of the oesophagus.
   d In the adventitial layer of the oesophagus.

73. The most common complication of Zenker's diverticulum is:
   a Dysphonia.
   b Gastro-oesophageal reflux.
   c Lung abscess.
   d Perforation.

74. The treatment of choice in a 50-year-old male with achalasia cardia is:
   a Laparoscopic Heller's cardiomyotomy.
   b Pneumatic balloon dilatation.
   c High-dose proton pump inhibitor.
   d Open Heller's cardiomyotomy.

75. The most common cause of gastroparesis is due to:
   a Diabetes.
   b Post-distal gastrectomy.
   c Post-vagotomy for ulcer disease.
   d Post-pancreaticoduodenectomy.

76. The following antacid preparation contains alginate:
    a Gaviscon.
    b Milk of magnesia.
    c Sucralfate.
    d Aluminium hydroxide.

77. The following drug reduces acid secretion by inhibiting histamine type 2 receptor:
    a Ranitidine.
    b Omeprazole.
    c Cisapride.
    d Gaviscon.

78. The long-term use of proton pump inhibitors can be associated with:
    a Gastric cancer.
    b Atrophic gastritis with intestinal metaplasia.
    c Carcinoid syndrome.
    d Cardiac arrhythmias.

79. The most frequent complication associated with anti-reflux surgery is:
    a Dysphagia.
    b Oesophageal perforation.
    c Failure to control reflux.
    d Injury to spleen.

80. Anti-reflux operations decrease the acid reflux by all of the following mechanisms, except:
    a Decreases the basal pressure generated by the lower oesophageal sphincter (LOS).
    b Exaggeration of the flap valve at the angle of His.
    c Reduction in the triggering of transient lower oesophageal sphincter relaxations.
    d Reduction in the capacity of the gastric fundus.

81. Anti-reflux surgery is not indicated in patients with:
    a Oesophageal stricture.
    b Reflux associated with chronic sinusitis.
    c Patients who failed to respond to medical therapy.
    d Patients who respond to medical treatment but do not want to continue life-long proton pump inhibitor.

82. The anti-reflux procedure described by Toupet is:
    a 270-degree posterior fundoplication.
    b 300-degree posterior fundoplication.
    c Anterior partial fundoplication.
    d Complete wrapping of the fundus of stomach around the lower oesophagus.

83. Which of the following statements regarding anti-reflux surgery is incorrect?
    a The division of short gastric vessels improves the outcome following Nissen fundoplication.
    b Partial fundoplication is associated with less wind-related problems than total fundoplication.
    c Nissen fundoplication has a lower complication and re-operation rate than the Angelchik prosthesis.
    d The inclusion or exclusion of the vagus nerve from the wrap makes no difference to the outcome.

84. A 30-year-old male underwent floppy Nissen fundoplication four hours ago. Post-operative chest X-ray showed pneumothorax on the left side. The patient is clinically well with normal oxygen saturation on 2 L of oxygen via nasal specs. The most appropriate treatment of pneumothorax is:
    a Insertion of chest drain.
    b Needle aspiration.
    c No further treatment.
    d Wait and watch and repeat chest X-ray in 24 hours.

85. The use of NSAIDs and aspirin is associated with duodenal and gastric ulcer formation. The mechanism of injury is due to:
    a Inhibition of cycloxygenase 1.
    b Inhibition of cycloxygenase 2.
    c Reduction in the production of bicarbonate.
    d Direct damage to the gastric and duodenal mucosa.

86. Which of the following statements regarding *Helicobacter pylori* infection is incorrect?
    a It is a spiral-shaped gram positive microaerophilic bacteria.
    b It is associated with duodenal and gastric ulcers.
    c It is the most common cause of non-NSAIDs-induced duodenal ulceration.
    d It can cause antral gastritis.

87. The ^{14}C urea breath test used in the detection of *Helicobacter pylori* infection is based on the production of which enzyme?
a Urease.
b Peroxidase.
c Hydroxylase.
d Dehydrogenase.

88. The following anti-ulcer agent works by inhibiting acid secretion and proteolytic enzymes, and increases bicarbonate and mucus secretion:
a Ranitidine.
b Misoprostol.
c Omeprazole.
d Cimitidine.

89. The condition that is not associated with high serum gastrin level is:
a Zollinger-Ellison syndrome.
b Pernicious anaemia.
c Long-term use of proton pump inhibitors.
d Long-term use of sucralfate.

90. A 35-year-old male patient presents with recurrent duodenal ulceration, diarrhoea and weight loss. Upper GI endoscopy reveals multiple duodenal ulcers. The most likely diagnosis is:
a Zollinger-Ellison syndrome.
b *Helicobacter pylori* infection.
c Insulinoma.
d VIPoma.

91. The most sensitive diagnostic test used for the detection of gastrinoma is:
a CT scan.
b Magnetic resonance imaging (MRI).
c Endoscopic ultrasound (EUS).
d Somatostatin receptor scintigraphy.

92. Which of the following statements regarding Zollinger-Ellison syndrome (ZES) is incorrect?
    a More than two-thirds of patients with ZES have other endocrine tumours.
    b Sporadic gastrinomas are associated with good prognosis.
    c The duodenum is the most common extrapancreatic site of gastrinoma.
    d Surgical resection of localised liver gastrinoma provides a cure rate similar to that of extrahepatic gastrinoma.

93. The preferred treatment of choice for the bleeding gastric ulcer at the incisura following failed endoscopic treatment is:
    a Under running of the bleeding ulcer.
    b Local excision of ulcer.
    c Partial gastrectomy.
    d Total gastrectomy.

94. The treatment of choice in a patient with a bleeding gastric ulcer high on the lesser curve is:
    a Total gastrectomy.
    b Local excision of the lesser curve.
    c Under running of the ulcer.
    d a or b.

95. A 25-year-old male patient presents with an upper GI bleed following heavy alcohol intake. The most likely cause of bleeding is:
    a Mallory–Weiss tear.
    b Spontaneous oesophageal perforation.
    c Gastric erosions.
    d Acute duodenal ulcer.

96. The most common site of spontaneous oesophageal perforation is:
    a Just below the upper oesophageal sphincter.
    b Just above the diaphragm in the left posterolateral position.
    c Just above the diaphragm in the right posterolateral position.
    d At the gastro-oesophageal junction.

97. A 45-year-old male patient presents with chest pain after a few episodes of vomiting following binge drinking over the weekend. On examination he looks unwell. His pulse rate is 90/min, BP normal and temperature 38°C. Chest X-ray shows pneumomediastinum and left-sided pleural effusion. The most likely diagnosis is:
    a   Boerhaave's syndrome.
    b   Perforated peptic ulcer.
    c   Mallory–Weiss tear.
    d   Spontaneous pneumothorax.

98. A 60-year-old female patient is referred by her general practitioner 48 hours after she underwent rigid oesophagoscopy and dilatation of a benign post-cricoid stricture. On admission, she is tachycardic with a pulse rate of 100/min, BP normal and temperature 38.5°C. Her white count is 15,000/mm³. An urgent CT chest and abdomen shows a contained leak. She should be managed with:
    a   Thoracotomy and washout and chest drain insertion.
    b   Thoracotomy, insertion of T-tube and chest tube insertion.
    c   Conservative treatment with antibiotics, antifungals and nil by mouth.
    d   Primary closure of oesophageal perforation, washout and chest drain insertion.

99. A 35-year-old male patient presents with severe chest pain following vomiting after binge drinking over the weekend. On examination, he is tachycardic, BP 90/60 mmHg, temperature 39°C and white count 13,000/mm³. His chest X-ray reveals air in the mediastinum. The appropriate treatment of choice is:
    a   Thoracotomy and washout and chest drain insertion.
    b   Thoracotomy, insertion of T-tube in the oesophageal perforation and chest tube insertion.
    c   Conservative treatment with antibiotics, antifungals and nil by mouth.
    d   Primary closure of oesophageal perforation, washout and chest drain insertion.

100. A 20-year-old female patient with full thickness oesophageal burn and perforation following ingestion of drain-cleaning fluid is admitted to the intensive care unit. She is intubated because of respiratory compromise and is started on broad spectrum antibiotics. The best surgical treatment option in this patient is:
   a Oesophagogastrectomy and immediate reconstruction with colonic interposition.
   b Oesophagogastrectomy and delayed reconstruction.
   c Cervical oesophagostomy, feeding jejunostomy and delayed resection and reconstruction.
   d Oesophagectomy and immediate reconstruction using gastric conduit.

101. The diagnostic investigation of choice in patients with suspected spontaneous oesophageal perforation is:
   a Oesophageal contrast study.
   b Upper GI endoscopy.
   c CT scan.
   d Chest X-ray.

102. Morbid obesity is when the body mass index (BMI) is greater than:
   a 30.
   b 35.
   c 40.
   d 45.

103. Which of the following conditions does not improve following bariatric surgery?
   a Obstructive sleep apnoea.
   b Diabetes mellitus.
   c Idiopathic intracranial hypertension.
   d Gastro-oesophageal reflux.
   e Chronic cholecystitis.

104. The pre-operative dietary measure that is used to reduce liver volume at the time of bariatric surgery is:
   a Low calorie diet for 6 weeks.
   b Very low calorie diet for 6 weeks.
   c Very low calorie and low protein diet for 6 weeks.
   d High carbohydrate and high protein diet for 6 weeks.

105. A 30-year-old female patient presents to A&E with severe dysphagia following gastric band surgery. The immediate step in the management of this patient is:
    a Laparoscopy and removal of gastric band.
    b Insertion of nasogastric tube.
    c Urgent gastroscopy and dilatation.
    d Deflation of gastric band reservoir.

106. The malabsorptive bariatric surgical procedure is:
    a Laparoscopic gastric banding.
    b Laparoscopic vertical banded gastroplasty.
    c Roux-en-Y gastric bypass.
    d Jejuno-ileal bypass.

107. All of the following are metabolic complications associated with morbid obesity, except:
    a Hypertension.
    b Dyslipidemia.
    c Diabetes mellitus.
    d Hypertrophic cardiomyopathy.

108. The ideal size of gastric pouch used in patients undergoing laparoscopic gastric banding is:
    a 5–10 cc.
    b 15–25 cc.
    c 50–60 cc.
    d 100–150 cc.

109. Which of the following bariatric surgical procedures is associated with a high improvement rate in diabetes, hypertension, hypercholesterolemia and sleep apnoea?
    a Vertical banded gastroplasty.
    b Gastric banding.
    c Roux-en-Y gastric bypass.
    d Biliary pancreatic diversion.

110. The side-effects of proton pump inhibitors include:
    a Headache.
    b Diarrhoea.
    c Constipation.
    d None of the above.
    e All of the above.

111. The risk of developing oesophageal carcinoma in Barrett's oesophagus is:
   a   0.5% per year.
   b   1% per year.
   c   5% per year.
   d   10% per year.

112. Dysphagia lusoria is due to:
   a   Oesophageal diverticulum.
   b   Aneurysm of the aorta.
   c   Oesophageal web.
   d   Compression by an aberrant blood vessel.

113. The most common type of tracheo-oesophageal fistula is:
   a   Proximal end blind, distal end communicating with the trachea.
   b   Distal end blind, proximal end communicating with the trachea.
   c   Both ends blind.
   d   Both ends open.

114. Which of the following conditions is the most likely diagnosis in
a neonate presenting with continuous dribbling of saliva from the
mouth?
   a   Oesophageal atresia.
   b   Duodenal atresia.
   c   Tracheo-oesophageal fistula.
   d   Anal atresia.

115. Which of the following statements regarding Zollinger-Ellison
syndrome is incorrect?
   a   It is associated with intractable peptic ulcers.
   b   It is associated with severe diarrhoea.
   c   It is a β-cell tumour of the pancreas.
   d   It is associated with high basal acid output.

116. All of the following features are associated with gastrinoma, except:
   a   Epigastric pain.
   b   Diarrhoea.
   c   Basal acid output (BAO) of less than 15 mEq/L.
   d   Serum gastrin level >200 pg/mL.

117. Raised gastrin levels without an associated increase in gastric acid secretions is seen in:
   a Gastric carcinoma.
   b Gastrinoma.
   c Pernicious anaemia.
   d G-cell hyperplasia.

118. The surgical method of choice for the treatment of duodenal atresia is:
   a Gastrojejunostomy.
   b Duodenojejunostomy/duodenoduodenostomy.
   c Partial gastrectomy.
   d Bishop-Koop operation.

Answers: Oesophagogastric surgery

1. d *Helicobacter pylori* infection.

2. a Adenocarcinoma.

3. b Middle third thoracic oesophagus.

4. a Hyperplastic polyps.

5. c Fundic gland polyp.

6. c Carcinoma limited to mucosa or submucosa irrespective of lymph node involvement.

7. a Ulcerating type (type III and IIc).

8. a They are predominantly found in the fundus of the stomach.

9. d E-cadherin.

10. a Stomach.

11. b Stomach.

12. a *Helicobacter pylori* eradication.

13. c 3 cm.

14. a Plummer-Vinson syndrome.

15. a Endoscopic ultrasound (EUS).

16. **d** All of the above.

17. **c** Gastric leiomyoma.

18. **a** It gives anatomical details of the tumour.

19. **e** PET-CT.

20. **b** Endoscopic ultrasound (EUS).

21. **b** Elongated, heterogenous, hyperechoic with indistinct borders.

22. **d** Lesser curvature near incisura angularis.

23. **d** All of the above.

24. **c** ASA-III.

25. **d** The functional capacity is considered excellent if METs are less than seven.

26. **d** a and b.

27. **a** Patients who had recent coronary artery bypass graft (CABG) surgery with good residual ventricular function.

28. **a** Who stop smoking 8 weeks before surgery.

29. **d** 5–10% of patients with pT1a have lymph node metastasis.

30. **b** Associated with higher risk of anastomotic leak.

31. **a** Stomach.

32. **c** Pneumonia.

33. **c** Chemoradiotherapy.

34. **b** It is an autosomal recessive disorder.

35. **c** Poorly-differentiated tumour.

36. a Aorta.

37. a T10.

38. a Mucosa.

39. a The azygous vein passes posterior to the oesophagus before joining the superior vena cava.

40. c Through posterior mediastinum.

41. d b and c.

42. d Right gastric artery and gastroepiploic arcade.

43. b Colon.

44. b In patients undergoing primary oesophageal resection.

45. b Lymphatics.

46. b It is more common in elderly patients.

47. d b and c.

48. d Stations 2 and 10.

49. d Stations 2 and 10.

50. d Station 12.

51. b Stations 2 and 10.

52. a Partial gastrectomy.

53. a Rapid movement of fluid into the small intestine from extra-
cellular fluid.

54. a Vitamin A, D and B12.

55. b They spread through the lymphatics.

56. a Presence of CD 117.

57. c Ki-67 proliferative index.

58. d High.

59. a Benign GISTs are more common in the small bowel.

60. c Positron emission tomography (PET)-CT.

61. c Wedge resection of the stomach.

62. a It blocks the binding of ATP to c-KIT.

63. b Resectable GIST.

64. a Presence of KIT exon 9 mutation.

65. a The lower third of the oesophagus is entirely composed of skeletal muscle.

66. d Diffuse oesophageal spasm.

67. b Inappropriate transient lower oesophageal sphincter relaxations.

68. a Presence of *Helicobacter pylori* infection is associated with increased acid secretion and GORD.

69. b 24-hour ambulatory pH monitoring.

70. a <4% of 24-hour period in normal individuals.

71. a Total acid reflux time.

72. a Between the outer longitudinal and inner circular muscle of the oesophagus.

73. c Lung abscess.

74. a Laparoscopic Heller's cardiomyotomy.

75. a Diabetes.

76. a Gaviscon.

77. a Ranitidine.

78. b Atrophic gastritis with intestinal metaplasia.

79. a Dysphagia.

80. a Decreases the basal pressure generated by the lower oesophageal sphincter (LOS).

81. a Oesophageal stricture.

82. a 270-degree posterior fundoplication.

83. a The division of short gastric vessels improves the outcome following Nissen fundoplication.

84. d Wait and watch and repeat chest X-ray in 24 hours.

85. a Inhibition of cycloxygenase 1.

86. a It is a spiral-shaped gram positive microaerophilic bacteria.

87. a Urease.

88. b Misoprostol.

89. d Long-term use of sucralfate.

90. a Zollinger-Ellison syndrome.

91. d Somatostatin receptor scintigraphy.

92. a More than two-thirds of patients with ZES have other endocrine tumours.

93. c Partial gastrectomy.

94. d a or b.

95. a Mallory–Weiss tear.

96. b Just above the diaphragm in the left posterolateral position.

97. a Boerhaave's syndrome.

98. c Conservative treatment with antibiotics, antifungals and nil by mouth.

99. b Thoracotomy, insertion of T-tube in the oesophageal perforation and chest tube insertion.

100. b Oesophagogastrectomy and delayed reconstruction.

101. a Oesophageal contrast study.

102. c 40.

103. e Chronic cholecystitis.

104. a Low calorie diet for 6 weeks.

105. d Deflation of gastric band reservoir.

106. d Jejuno-ileal bypass.

107. d Hypertrophic cardiomyopathy.

108. b 15–25 cc.

109. d Biliary pancreatic diversion.

110. e All of the above.

111. a 0.5% per year.

112. d Compression by an aberrant blood vessel.

113. a Proximal end blind, distal end communicating with the trachea.

114. a Oesophageal atresia.

115. c It is a β-cell tumour of the pancreas.

116. c Basal acid output (BAO) of less than 15 mEq/L.

117. c Pernicious anaemia.

118. b Duodenojejunostomy/duodenoduodenostomy.

4
Hepatobiliary and pancreatic surgery

Questions

1. The anatomical division of the liver is based on:
   a Hepatic artery and bile duct anatomy.
   b Surface markings of the liver.
   c Portal vein and hepatic artery anatomy.
   d Hepatic artery, hepatic vein and biliary anatomy.

✓ 2. Which of the following statements regarding the anatomy of the liver is true?
   a The anatomical division of the hepatic artery, bile duct and portal vein is regular and identical.
   b The hepatic artery and bile duct anatomy is regular and identical.
   c The hepatic artery and portal vein anatomy is regular and identical.
   d The bile duct and portal vein anatomy is regular and identical.

3. Anatomically the liver can be divided into:
   a 4 sectors and 9 segments.
   b 6 sectors and 9 segments.
   c 5 sectors and 9 segments.
   d 8 sectors and 8 segments.

4. Which of the following statements regarding the plane that intersects the liver into the right and left liver is true?
   a It goes through the falciform ligament.
   b It goes through the inferior vena cava and gallbladder.
   c It goes through the right hepatic vein.
   d It goes through the left hepatic vein.

5. Which one of the following statements regarding the volume of the normal liver is true?
    a The ratio between the right and left liver is 40:60.
    b The ratio between the right and left liver is 60:40.
    c The ratio between the right and left liver is 50:50.
    d The ratio between the right and left liver is 75:25.

6. Which one of the following statements with regard to the histology of the liver is incorrect?
    a A lobule is the basic functional unit of the liver.
    b Liver sinusoids are lined by endothelial cells and Kupffer cells.
    c The central part of the liver lobule has a better supply of oxygen and nutrients.
    d The portal triad consists of branches of the portal vein, hepatic artery and bile duct.

7. Which of the following statements regarding the caudate lobe of the liver is true?
    a It receives its arterial supply from the right hepatic artery.
    b It receives its arterial supply from both the right and left hepatic arteries.
    c It drains into the right hepatic vein.
    d It drains into the left hepatic duct.

8. Which of the following statements regarding the anatomy of the left branch of the portal vein is true?
    a It acts as a conduit between the umbilical vein and ductus venosus *in utero*.
    b It has horizontal and transverse portions.
    c The horizontal portion is located under segment 4.
    d All of the above.

9. The ligamentum venosum is:
    a A remnant of the ductus venosus.
    b Obliterated left umbilical artery.
    c Obliterated right umbilical vein.
    d A remnant of the vitellointestinal duct.

10. Which of the following statements regarding the anatomy of the left hepatic vein is true?
    a It begins in the plane between segments 2 and 4.
    b It begins in the plane between segments 2 and 3.
    c It joins the right hepatic vein before it joins the inferior vena cava.
    d The umbilical vein attaches to the left hepatic vein at its insertion into the inferior vena cava.

11. Which of the following statements regarding the anatomical importance of the cystic plate is true?
    a It attaches directly on to the anterior surface of the right portal pedicle.
    b It must be divided to visualise the anterior surface of the right portal pedicle.
    c It is the fibrous surface that is encountered during cholecystectomy.
    d All of the above.

12. The most posterior structure in the hepatoduodenal ligament is:
    a Hepatic artery.
    b Portal vein.
    c Common bile duct.
    d Inferior vena cava.

13. Which one of the following statements regarding the arterial supply of the liver is true?
    a A replaced artery means that it is an additional artery supplying the liver.
    b In the majority of patients the right hepatic artery originates from the superior mesenteric artery.
    c In 25% of patients part or all of the liver is supplied by a replaced artery.
    d The left hepatic artery originates from the left gastric artery.

14. The most common anatomical variation of the portal vein is:
    a Absence of the right portal vein.
    b Absence of the left portal vein.
    c Absence of the right posterior sectional vein.
    d Absence of the left medial sectional vein.

15. The boundaries of the hepatocystic (Calot's) triangle are formed by the:
    a Right side of the common hepatic duct, liver and cystic duct.
    b Gallbladder, common bile duct and liver.
    c Gallbladder, cystic artery and cystic duct.
    d Gallbladder, right hepatic artery and right hepatic duct.

16. All of the following are the contents of the hepatocystic (Calot's) triangle, except:
    a Cystic artery.
    b Cystic lymph node.
    c A portion of the right hepatic artery.
    d Cystic duct.

17. The arterial supply to the bile duct is derived from:
    a The portion of the bile duct below the bifurcation and above the duodenum is supplied by two longitudinal arteries at the 3 and 9 o'clock positions.
    b The portion of the bile duct below the bifurcation and above the duodenum is supplied by two longitudinal arteries at the 6 and 12 o'clock positions.
    c The lower end of the bile duct is supplied by the gastroduodenal artery.
    d a and c.
    e b and c.

18. To avoid injury to the pancreatic duct during sphincteroplasty, the ampulla of Vater should be opened between:
    a 10 and 12 o'clock.
    b 12 and 2 o'clock.
    c 9 and 6 o'clock.
    d 4 and 6 o'clock.

19. Which one of the following structures is not related to the posterior surface of the pancreas?
    a Right kidney.
    b Inferior vena cava and right gonadal vein.
    c Abdominal aorta.
    d Right adrenal gland.

20. The most common benign liver tumour of mesenchymal origin is:
    a Haemangioma.
    b Liver cell adenoma.
    c Biliary cystadenoma.
    d Focal nodular hyperplasia.

21. Which of the following statements regarding haemangioma of the liver is true?
    a Cavernous haemangioma is more common than capillary haemangioma.
    b Cavernous haemangiomas are small and often multiple.
    c There is usually a normal plane between the haemangioma and liver tissue.
    d Haemangiomas are usually symptomatic.

22. The most accurate test in the diagnosis and characterisation of cavernous haemangioma of the liver is:
    a Computed tomography of the liver.
    b Ultrasound of the liver.
    c Magnetic resonance imaging of the liver.
    d Doppler ultrasound of the liver.

23. In patients with haemangioma of the liver, surgery should be offered to patients with:
    a Symptomatic lesion.
    b Haemangioma of more than 4 cm.
    c Haemangioma of more than 10 cm.
    d Small haemangioma with abdominal pain.

24. All of the following increases the risk of liver cell adenoma, except:
    a Androgen steroids.
    b Diabetes.
    c Glycogen storage diseases.
    d Tyrosinaemia.

25. Which of the following statements regarding liver cell adenoma is true?
    a They are usually multiple.
    b Liver cell adenoma infrequently presents with pain due to haemorrhage.
    c It is associated with an increased risk of haemorrhage during pregnancy.
    d It is common in males.

26. Which one of the following statements regarding treatment of liver cell adenoma is correct?
    a Surgery should be considered in all patients.
    b Surgery should be considered only in symptomatic patients.
    c Surgery should be considered only in patients with haemorrhage.
    d Surgery should be considered only in patients with multiple lesions.

27. Focal nodular hyperplasia is:
    a A pre-malignant tumour.
    b Associated with oral contraceptive usage.
    c Associated with intralesional haemorrhage.
    d A benign liver lesion.

28. Which one of the following statements regarding the management of focal nodular hyperplasia is correct?
    a It does not require surgery.
    b It should be resected in all cases.
    c It should be resected only if there is a diagnostic uncertainty.
    d None of the above.

29. The most commonly isolated organisms from a pyogenic liver abscess are:
    a *Escherichia coli, Klebsiella, Bacteroides.*
    b *Pseudomonas aeruginosa.*
    c *Streptococcus faecalis.*
    d *Staphylococcus aureus.*

30. The most common aetiology of liver abscess is:
    a Cholangitis.
    b Appendicitis.
    c Diverticulitis.
    d Pneumonia.

31. A 65-year-old male patient presents with gallstones and a 7 cm liver abscess adjacent to the gallbladder. The most appropriate treatment is:
   a Cholecystectomy followed by 3–6 week course of antibiotics.
   b Percutaneous drainage of the liver abscess and interval cholecystectomy.
   c Percutaneous aspiration of the liver abscess and interval cholecystectomy.
   d A long course of antibiotics.

32. An 'anchovy sauce' appearance of fluid aspirated from a liver abscess is characteristic of:
   a Pyogenic liver abscess.
   b Amoebic liver abscess.
   c Infected hydatid cyst.
   d Necrotic liver metastasis.

33. All of the following are intermediate hosts for *Echinococcus* infection, except:
   a Dogs.
   b Sheep.
   c Humans.
   d Goats.

34. Cystadenoma of the liver is a:
   a Pre-malignant tumour.
   b Benign tumour.
   c Malignant tumour.
   d None of the above.

35. The treatment of choice for cystadenoma of liver is:
   a Surgical excision in all patients.
   b Surgical excision if there are any features suggestive of malignancy on imaging.
   c Surgery should be offered to symptomatic patients.
   d No treatment required.

36. Which one of the following statements regarding the aetiology of hepatocellular carcinoma of the liver is not true?
   a It can develop at any stage of hepatitis B infection.
   b It is very rare in patients with hepatitis C without cirrhosis.
   c It can develop in patients with hepatitis E infection.
   d None of the above.

37. All of the following are risk factors for hepatocellular carcinoma (HCC), except:
   a Hepatitis B infection.
   b Oral contraceptive usage.
   c Hepatitis C infection.
   d Obesity.

38. The risk of hepatocellular carcinoma (HCC) is low in which one of the following groups of patients with hepatitis B infection:
   a HBsAg and HBeAg positive patients.
   b HBsAg negative patients.
   c Alcohol and alfatoxin exposure.
   d HBsAg antibody positive patients.

39. The best and the most effective way of decreasing the incidence of hepatitis B virus (HBV) related hepatocellular carcinoma (HCC) is:
   a Vaccination against hepatitis B virus.
   b Regular exercise and avoiding alcohol.
   c Hepatitis B immunoglobulin injection on a regular basis.
   d Anti-retroviral medication.

40. The risk of hepatocellular carcinoma (HCC) correlates with:
   a Age.
   b Male gender.
   c Duration of disease.
   d Severity of hepatitis.
   e All of the above.

41. Which one of the following statements regarding hepatitis C virus (HCV) related hepatocellular carcinoma (HCC) is true?
   a HCC can be seen in patients without cirrhosis.
   b HCV related HCC is very rare before the age of 40 in the absence of other co-factors.
   c The risk of HCC is high in females.
   d The risk of HCC is not related to the duration of disease.

42. All of the following are risk factors for hepatocellular carcinoma (HCC), except:
   a Haemochromatosis.
   b Tay-Sachs disease.
   c α-1 antitrypsin deficiency.
   d Non-alcoholic fatty liver disease.

43. In patients with hepatocellular carcinoma (HCC), portal vein invasion is influenced by all of the following factors, except:
   a Gender.
   b Type of HCC.
   c Differentiation of the tumour.
   d Size of the tumour.

44. The most common site of metastases in patients with hepatocellular carcinoma (HCC) is:
   a Adrenal gland.
   b Bone.
   c Lymph node.
   d Lungs.

45. A 60-year-old male patient of Asian origin with a known history of cirrhosis of the liver presents to A&E with a sudden onset of severe epigastric pain. On clinical examination he is pale, pulse rate 110/min and blood pressure 100/50 mmHg. Abdominal examination reveals signs of peritonitis. What is the most likely diagnosis?
   a Ruptured hepatocellular carcinoma (HCC).
   b Acute pancreatitis.
   c Perforated duodenal ulcer.
   d Perforated diverticular disease.

46. Which of the following statements regarding α-fetoprotein (AFP) as a tumour marker for hepatocellular carcinoma (HCC) is true?
   a AFP has high sensitivity and specificity.
   b 75% of patients with chronic active hepatitis without HCC can have a raised AFP.
   c AFP has low sensitivity and specificity.
   d AFP is also elevated in other tumours.

47. The characteristic feature of hepatocellular carcinoma (HCC) on contrast enhanced CT scan is:
  a Late uptake and late washout.
  b Early uptake and early washout.
  c Early uptake and late washout.
  d A hyperdense lesion with extrahepatic lymph node involvement.

48. The investigation of choice for the diagnosis of hepatocellular carcinoma (HCC) of size less than 2 cm is:
  a Ultrasound.
  b CT scan.
  c Magnetic resonance imaging of the liver.
  d Contrast ultrasound.

49. Screening should be considered for a disease:
  a When the mortality from the disease is very high.
  b When there is no clearly defined progression of the disease from pre-malignant to malignant lesions.
  c When there is no available diagnostic tool to diagnose the disease early.
  d When early diagnosis doesn't affect patient survival.

50. The treatment of choice in patients with a 4 cm hepatocellular carcinoma (HCC) in a non-cirrhotic liver is:
  a Liver transplantation.
  b Liver resection.
  c Chemoembolisation.
  d Percutaneous ethanol injection.

51. The best treatment option for a 3 cm nodule suspicious of hepatocellular carcinoma (HCC) in a 40-year-old male patient with Child's A cirrhosis is:
  a Radiofrequency ablation.
  b Liver transplantation.
  c Transarterial chemoembolisation (TACE).
  d TACE followed by liver transplantation.

52. Liver transplantation is inappropriate in all of the following scenarios, except:
    a 5 cm suspicious nodule in a cirrhotic liver.
    b 5 suspicious nodules each measuring less than 4.5 cm.
    c Child's C cirrhosis with a suspicious nodule of 8 cm.
    d Multiple suspicious nodules each measuring less than 1 cm.

53. All of the following variables have been found to be associated with an increased risk of recurrence of hepatocellular carcinoma (HCC), except:
    a Presence of capsular invasion.
    b Tumour >5 cm.
    c Presence of venous invasion.
    d Intra-operative blood transfusion.

54. The rationale behind the use of transarterial chemoembolisation (TACE) as one of the treatment options for hepatocellular carcinoma (HCC) is:
    a It receives blood supply from the hepatic artery.
    b It receives blood supply from the portal vein.
    c It is the most effective treatment.
    d It affects lesions which are not visualised by either CT or magnetic resonance imaging of the liver.

55. All of the following are contraindications for transarterial chemoembolisation (TACE), except:
    a Decompensated liver disease.
    b Gallstones.
    c Biliary obstruction.
    d Portal vein thrombosis.

56. Complications of transarterial chemoembolisation (TACE) include:
    a Chemoembolisation syndrome.
    b Acute cholecystitis.
    c Duodenal perforation.
    d Acute pancreatitis.
    e All of the above.

57. The fibrolamellar variant of hepatocellular carcinoma (HCC) differs from classical HCC in all of the following factors, except:
   a It is associated with good prognosis.
   b It is more common in females.
   c It occurs at a young age.
   d It is uncommon in patients with chronic liver disease.

58. The characteristic of colorectal liver metastases on CT scan is:
   a Hypervascular.
   b Hypovascular.
   c Hyperdense.
   d Calcification.

59. A 35-year-old male patient with a right-sided colonic carcinoma is found to have multiple colorectal liver metastases confined to the right liver by staging CT. This patient should be offered:
   a Right hemicolectomy followed by right hepatectomy.
   b Liver resection followed by right hemicolectomy at a later stage.
   c Simultaneous right hemicolectomy and right hepatectomy.
   d Neoadjuvant chemotherapy followed by liver and colonic resection.

60. Liver resection is not indicated in patients with which of the following:
   a 5 cm metastatic deposit in the left lateral sector.
   b 3 cm metastatic deposit in the right posterior sector.
   c Unresectable extrahepatic lymph nodal disease.
   d 3 cm metastatic deposit in the right lower lobe of the lung.

61. Autoimmune pancreatitis is associated with elevated serum levels of which of the following immunoglobulins (Ig)?
   a IgG4.
   b IgM.
   c IgA.
   d IgD.

62. The treatment of choice for patients with suspected autoimmune pancreatitis is:
   a Steroids.
   b NSAIDs.
   c Infliximab.
   d Methotrexate.

63. Which of the following statements regarding gallbladder dyskinesia is incorrect?
   a It is associated with abnormal liver enzymes.
   b It is associated with the absence of sludge, stones or microlithiasis in the gallbladder.
   c The gallbladder ejection fraction after infusion of cholecystokinin for more than 30 minutes is less than 40%.
   d Pain is not relieved by bowel movements, postural change or antacids.

64. Which of the following is not an effect of cholecystokinin?
   a Relaxation of the sphincter of Oddi.
   b Relaxation of the pylorus.
   c Contraction of the gallbladder.
   d Relaxation of the lower oesophageal sphincter.

65. The gold standard test used in the diagnosis of dysfunction of the sphincter of Oddi is:
   a Manometry.
   b Endoscopic retrograde pancreaticography (ERCP).
   c Endoscopic ultrasound (EUS).
   d Cholecystokinin scintigraphy.

66. Which of the following statements regarding type 1 dysfunction of the sphincter of Oddi is incorrect?
   a Usually requires manometry to establish the diagnosis.
   b Manometry can be normal in 14–35% of patients.
   c Over 90% benefit from sphincterotomy.
   d Associated with a common bile duct diameter of more than 8 mm.

67. Which one of the following is not required for making a diagnosis of pancreatic sphincter of Oddi dysfunction (SOD)?
   a Normal pancreatic enzymes.
   b Pancreatic enzymes >1.5 times normal.
   c Pancreatic duct diameter of more than 6 mm in the neck and >5 mm in the body.
   d Delayed drainage of contrast by ERCP of >9 min.

68. Which of the following statements regarding capecitabine is incorrect?
    a It is an analogue of 5-fluorouracil (5-FU).
    b It acts by inhibiting thymidine phosphorylase.
    c It is as effective as 5-FU.
    d It is the oral form of 5-FU.

69. A 56-year-old male patient with neurofibromatosis presents with right renal cell carcinoma with involvement of the adrenal gland and segments V and VI of the liver. The best treatment option is:
    a Chemotherapy followed by surgery.
    b Right radical nephrectomy and right hemihepatectomy.
    c Palliative chemotherapy.
    d Chemoradiotherapy followed by radical nephrectomy and liver resection.

70. The side-effects of oxaliplatin include all of the following, except:
    a Blue liver syndrome.
    b Peripheral neuropathy.
    c Hand-foot syndrome.
    d None of the above.

71. Which of the following factors is not useful in predicting the risk of variceal haemorrhage?
    a Aetiology of the cirrhosis.
    b Size of the varices.
    c Severity of liver dysfunction.
    d Presence of red spots or a red wheal on oesophagogastroscopy.

72. Which of the following parameters are included in the Child–Pugh scoring system?
    a Bilirubin, albumin, prothrombin time, ascites and nutritional status.
    b Bilirubin, albumin, prothrombin time, ascites and encephalopathy.
    c Bilirubin, creatinine, prothrombin time, ascites and nutritional status.
    d Bilirubin, sodium, prothrombin time, ascites and nutritional status.

73. The risk of early variceal re-haemorrhage is increased by all of the following factors, except:
   a A hepatic venous pressure gradient of >12 mmHg.
   b Active haemorrhage at the time of initial endoscopy.
   c Presence of ascites.
   d None of the above.

74. The incidence of re-haemorrhage from oesophageal varices in the first 6 weeks is:
   a 5%.
   b 10–15%.
   c 30–40%.
   d 75%.

75. Which of the following parameters are included in the calculation of the modified end-stage liver disease (MELD) scoring system?
   a Sodium, international normalised ratio (INR), bilirubin and creatinine.
   b INR, bilirubin and creatinine.
   c Bilirubin, albumin, prothrombin time, ascites and encephalopathy.
   d Bilirubin, albumin, prothrombin time, ascites and nutritional status.

76. All of the following except one is an extrahepatic cause of portal hypertension:
   a Schistosomiasis.
   b Portal vein thrombosis.
   c Splenic vein thrombosis.
   d Tropical splenomegaly.

77. The Child–Pugh score in a 35-year-old male patient with alcoholic cirrhosis, with a moderate amount of ascites, normal sensorium, bilirubin of 35 mmol/L, albumin of 30 gm/L and prothrombin time of 23 seconds is:
   a 5.
   b 7.
   c 8.
   d 9.

78. In patients with portal hypertension, the appearance of complications such as variceal haemorrhage and ascites occur when the hepatic venous pressure gradient is greater than:
    a 5 mmHg.
    b 12 mmHg.
    c 20 mmHg.
    d 5 mmH$_2$O.

79. The best prophylactic option in preventing a variceal bleed in a patient who cannot tolerate β-blockers is:
    a Therapy with nitrate.
    b Distal splenorenal shunt.
    c Variceal sclerotherapy.
    d Variceal band ligation.

80. The treatment of choice to stop variceal bleed following initial resuscitation is:
    a Endoscopic sclerotherapy.
    b Endoscopic band ligation.
    c Injection of adrenaline.
    d Transjugular portosystemic shunt.

81. The initial treatment of choice in a patient presenting with haemorrhage from gastric varices is:
    a Endoscopic sclerotherapy with cyanoacrylate.
    b Variceal band ligation.
    c Sengsten–Blakemore tube intubation.
    d Transjugular portosystemic shunt.

82. The risk of encephalopathy is greater following transjugular intrahepatic portosystemic shunt (TIPS) procedure in patients with:
    a Advanced liver disease.
    b Patients with a prior history of encephalopathy.
    c Younger patients.
    d Patients with small diameter shunts.

83. The best treatment option for a patient with cirrhosis with refractory ascites is:
    a Repeated large volume paracentesis.
    b Transjugular intrahepatic portosystemic shunt (TIPS).
    c Sapheno-peritoneal shunt.
    d Liver transplantation.

84. Budd–Chiari syndrome occurs due to:
    a Occlusion of the hepatic veins.
    b Cirrhosis of the liver.
    c Occlusion of the portal vein.
    d Occlusion of the splenic vein.

85. All of the following are clinical features of acute Budd–Chiari syndrome, except:
    a Acute abdominal pain.
    b Abdominal swelling.
    c Acute fulminant liver failure.
    d Oesophageal variceal haemorrhage.

86. The most useful surrogate marker of the optimum dose of β-blockers in the absence of a hepatic venous pressure gradient measurement for the primary prophylaxis of variceal haemorrhage is:
    a Clinical tolerance.
    b Heart rate decreases by 25%.
    c Arterial hypotension.
    d Development of asthma.

87. The treatment of choice in a patient with acute Budd–Chiari syndrome not responding to medical treatment is:
    a Transjugular intrahepatic portosystemic shunt (TIPS).
    b Shunt surgery.
    c Liver transplantation.
    d Transjugular or transfemoral balloon dilatation of the hepatic vein.

88. The treatment of choice in a patient with segmental left-sided portal hypertension due to splenic vein thrombosis secondary to chronic pancreatitis is:
    a Transjugular intrahepatic portosystemic shunt (TIPS).
    b No specific treatment required.
    c Liver transplantation.
    d Splenectomy.

89. The following vaccines are recommended following splenectomy:
    a Pneumococcal, *H influenzae*, meningococcal.
    b Hepatitis B, pneumococcal, meningococcal.
    c Pneumococcal, hepatitis A, meningococcal.
    d Meningococcal, Japanese encephalitis, hepatitis B.

90. In the majority of cases, overwhelming post-splenectomy infection (OPSI) is due to:
    a *Streptococcus pneumoniae.*
    b *Haemophilus influenzae.*
    c *Capnocytophaga canimorsus.*
    d *Escherichia coli.*

91. A 14-year-old boy was chased by his friends and hit by a large stone on his left lower chest and renal angle. He managed to get home and was found collapsed in his bedroom by his mother. At the time of his arrival to A&E, his GCS is 13/15, pulse 130/min, systolic blood pressure 80 mmHg, and on clinical examination he has tenderness over his left renal angle and left upper quadrant. Chest X-rays show a fracture of the 9th and 10th ribs. The initial management of this patient includes:
    a Urgent CT scan of the abdomen.
    b Focused abdominal sonography for trauma (FAST) scan.
    c Fluid resuscitation.
    d Laparotomy.

92. The indication for angiography in haemodynamically stable patients with splenic trauma include all of the following, except:
    a Grade 1 and 2 injury.
    b Grade 3 or higher injury.
    c Evidence of ongoing haemorrhage on CT scan.
    d Presence of pseudoaneurysm.

93. The most common type of gallstones are:
    a Mixed cholesterol and pigment stones.
    b Pigment stones.
    c Cholesterol stones.
    d Calcium oxalate stones.

94. A 25-year-old female patient presents with acute lower chest pain associated with vomiting. Her pulse rate is 90/min and temperature 37.5°C. Clinical examination reveals mild tenderness in the right upper quadrant. An ultrasound scan shows gallstones. She is treated with analgesics and discharged home with a date for elective laparoscopic cholecystectomy. She represents a week later with features of obstructive jaundice. What is the next step in the management of this case?
    a Endoscopic retrograde cholangiopancreatography (ERCP) and extraction of the bile duct stones.
    b Repeat ultrasound scan.
    c Laparoscopic cholecystectomy with bile duct exploration.
    d Open cholecystectomy with bile duct exploration.

95. All of the following are risk factors for cholesterol gallstones, except:
    a Haemolytic anaemia.
    b Cirrhosis.
    c Diabetes mellitus.
    d Long-term parenteral nutrition.

96. The pathogenesis of cholesterol stones is due to:
    a Loss of equilibrium between cholesterol, bile pigments and the water content of bile.
    b Loss of equilibrium between phospholipids, cholesterol and bile salts.
    c Bacterial infection of bile.
    d An excessive amount of cholesterol in diet.

97. The most sensitive and specific test for the detection of gallstones in the bile duct is:
    a Magnetic resonance cholangiopancreatography (MRCP).
    b Endoscopic ultrasound (EUS).
    c Ultrasound scan.
    d CT scan.

98. Bile acids are the end products of:
    a Cholesterol metabolism.
    b Bilirubin metabolism.
    c Bile salts metabolism.
    d Lecithin metabolism.

99. A 55-year-old female patient with a history of previous laparotomy for necrotising pancreatitis and an open cholecystectomy presents with obstructive jaundice. Ultrasound confirms a dilated bile duct and a stone in the lower end of the bile duct. What is the best treatment option for this patient?

    a Magnetic resonance cholangiopancreatography (MRCP) followed by endoscopic retrograde cholangiopancreatography if the stone is confirmed on MRCP.

    b Open bile duct exploration.

    c Laparoscopic bile duct exploration.

    d Endoscopic retrograde cholangiopancreatography and stone extraction.

100. A 45-year-old male patient is investigated by his general practitioner for non-specific upper abdominal pain. An ultrasound scan shows a 0.5 cm single, non-mobile lesion in the gallbladder highly suggestive of a gallbladder polyp. The treatment of choice is:

    a Laparoscopic cholecystectomy.

    b Open cholecystectomy.

    c Reassurance.

    d Further imaging with CT scan.

101. A 50-year-old female with a body mass index (BMI) of 42 and a history of hypertension and type II diabetes, presents with symptomatic gallstones. She is seen by a general surgeon who proposes laparoscopic cholecystectomy. However, she is quite keen to have both weight loss surgery and cholecystectomy at the same time. Which one of the following statements regarding her further management is correct?

    a She should just undergo laparoscopic cholecystectomy.

    b She should be considered for laparoscopic banding and cholecystectomy at the same time.

    c She should undergo cholecystectomy followed by laparoscopic banding at a later date.

    d She should be considered for laparoscopic bypass followed by laparoscopic cholecystectomy at a later date.

102. The gold standard diagnostic tool used for the diagnosis of extra-hepatic biliary atresia is:
    a Preoperative cholangiography.
    b Hepatobiliary scintigraphy.
    c MRI of the liver.
    d Liver biopsy.

103. A 17-year-old female presents with upper abdominal pain, fever, jaundice and a palpable abdominal mass. The most likely diagnosis is:
    a Gallstone with cholangitis.
    b Mirizzi's syndrome.
    c Choledochal cyst.
    d Acute cholecystitis.

104. The treatment of choice in a patient with type I, II and III choledochal cyst is:
    a Cystoenterostomy.
    b Complete excision of the cyst followed by Roux-en-Y hepatico-jejunostomy.
    c Further treatment is not required if the patient is not symptomatic.
    d Partial cyst excision.

105. All of the following are complications of choledochal cyst, except:
    a Obstructive jaundice.
    b Pancreatic carcinoma.
    c Cholangitis.
    d Cholangiocarcinoma.

106. A 25-year-old female underwent a day case laparoscopic cholecystectomy for gallstones. She was discharged home on the same day. However, she is admitted the following day with severe abdominal pain. On examination, her pulse rate is 110/min and her temperature 38°C. Abdominal examination reveals tenderness in the right upper abdomen. Her white cell count is 13,000/mm³ and liver function tests are normal. The most likely diagnosis is:
    a Right lower lobe pneumonia.
    b Common bile duct stone.
    c Bile leak.
    d Acute pancreatitis.

107. A 40-year-old female patient underwent laparoscopic cholecystectomy, which was complicated by haemorrhage that was managed appropriately during the laparoscopic procedure. 24 hours later she becomes acutely unwell with signs of localised right upper quadrant peritonitis. The most appropriate management of this includes:

a Urgent ultrasound of abdomen.

b Consider repeat laparoscopy and washout.

c Consider laparotomy.

d Fluid resuscitation followed by endoscopic retrograde cholangiopancreatography (ERCP).

108. A 25-year-old female is readmitted with severe abdominal pain 24 hours following laparoscopic cholecystectomy. She is taken back to the operating theatre for a repeat laparoscopy. At laparoscopy, a large amount of bile is present in the right upper quadrant. The most common cause of bile leak following laparoscopic cholecystectomy is:

a Cystic duct stump leak.

b Bile leak from the duct of Luschka.

c Bile duct injury.

d Perforated duodenum with a bile leak.

109. A 30-year-old female is readmitted with acute abdominal pain 24 hours after laparoscopic cholecystectomy. On clinical examination she is jaundiced with a pulse rate of 100/min and temperature of 37.5°C. Abdominal examination reveals tenderness in the right upper quadrant. Her bilirubin is 80 mmol/L and alkaline phosphatase (ALP) 1618 IU/L. Ultrasound of the abdomen could not visualise the bile duct due to gas in the bowel. An urgent endoscopic retrograde cholangiopancreatography (ERCP) showed complete obstruction at the level of mid-common bile duct. Which one of the following is the best treatment option regarding further management of this case?

a Early repair of the bile duct by a general surgeon.

b Early repair of the bile duct by a hepatobiliary and pancreatic surgeon.

c Late repair of the bile duct by a hepatobiliary and pancreatic surgeon.

d PTC and stenting followed by delayed repair of the bile duct.

110. The predictors of a poor outcome following repair of the bile duct after bile duct injury are:
    a Repair by the injuring surgeon.
    b Vascular injury.
    c Involvement of biliary confluence.
    d All of the above.

111. The most common site of biliary tract cancer is:
    a Intrahepatic biliary tree.
    b Confluence of biliary tree.
    c Extrahepatic bile duct.
    d Gallbladder.

112. The most common site of cholangiocarcinoma is:
    a Hilum.
    b Intrahepatic.
    c Distal bile duct.
    d Gallbladder.

113. All of the following are risk factors for cholangiocarcinoma, except:
    a Primary sclerosing cholangitis.
    b Previous endoscopic sphincterotomy.
    c Choledochal cyst.
    d Gallstones.

114. Which one of the following is not a risk factor for cholangiocarcinoma?
    a Ulcerative colitis.
    b Clonorchis sinensis.
    c Choledochal cyst.
    d Chronic pancreatitis.

115. Which of the following statements regarding the prognosis of chol-angiocarcinoma is true?
    a Sclerosing type is associated with an excellent prognosis.
    b Papillary type is associated with a poor prognosis.
    c Nodular sclerosing type is associated with a good prognosis.
    d Papillary type is associated with a good prognosis.

116. Which of the following statements regarding the management of cholangiocarcinoma is not correct?
   a It is often difficult to make a diagnosis based on biopsy results.
   b The diagnosis of cholangiocarcinoma is mainly based on radiological investigation.
   c Distal cholangiocarcinomas have a better prognosis than hilar cholangiocarcinomas.
   d It is essential to make a histological diagnosis before treatment.

117. Which of the following is the most likely diagnosis in a 70-year-old male patient with painless obstructive jaundice associated with significant weight loss and a palpable gallbladder?
   a Hilar cholangiocarcinoma.
   b Common bile duct (CBD) stones.
   c Carcinoma of the head of the pancreas.
   d Duodenal carcinoma.

118. In patients with suspected cholangiocarcinoma, the presence of lobar atrophy indicates:
   a A locally advanced lesion.
   b An unresectable lesion.
   c Involvement of the hepatic artery.
   d Involvement of the portal vein.
   e a and d.

119. In patients with suspected resectable cholangiocarcinoma, percutaneous and endoscopic intervention should be avoided before surgery due to:
   a Risk of needle tract seeding following percutaneous intervention.
   b Risk of cholangitis.
   c Risk of pancreatitis.
   d Risk of haemorrhage.

120. All of the following criteria indicate an unresectable cholangiocarcinoma, except:
   a Cirrhosis of the liver.
   b Tumour extending into secondary radicals on both sides.
   c Tumour involving the biliary confluence.
   d Tumour involving the main portal vein proximal to its bifurcation.

121. Which of the following statements regarding the treatment of hilar cholangiocarcinoma is incorrect?
    a Resection is the most effective therapy.
    b R_0 resection is associated with good prognosis.
    c Partial hepatectomy is almost always necessary to achieve a tumour-free margin.
    d Caudate lobe resection is not associated with improved negative margins.

122. The independent predictors of long-term survival following surgery for hilar cholangiocarcinoma include all, except:
    a R_0 resection.
    b Concomitant liver resection.
    c Poorly-differentiated histology.
    d Papillary tumour type.

123. A 55-year-old male patient was recently diagnosed with hilar cholangiocarcinoma with atrophy of the right lobe of the liver. He was also found to have main portal vein involvement. He is discussed in a multidisciplinary meeting and it is decided to palliate his jaundice. The best palliative procedure is:
    a Percutaneous drainage of the left ductal system.
    b Percutaneous drainage of the right ductal system.
    c Endoscopic drainage.
    d Surgical bypass.

124. The risk of gallbladder cancer is high in all of the following conditions, except:
    a Gallbladder polyp >1 cm.
    b Cholecystoenteric fistula.
    c Porcelain gallbladder.
    d Previous endoscopic sphincterotomy.

125. Cholecystectomy is indicated in all of the following conditions, except:
    a Patients with a gallbladder polyp >1 cm in diameter.
    b Patients with a carcinoid tumour requiring small bowel resection.
    c Patients with asymptomatic gallstones.
    d Patients with a porcelain gallbladder.

126. The indications for cholecystectomy in patients with asymptomatic gallstones include all, except:
    a   Patients with cirrhosis.
    b   Patients waiting for heart transplantation.
    c   Patients with type II diabetes.
    d   Patients with a porcelain gallbladder.

127. A 50-year-old female patient of Asian origin was recently diagnosed with gallbladder cancer with the involvement of the hepatic flexure and the second part of the duodenum. The stage for this tumour is:
    a T_2.
    b T_3.
    c T_{1b}.
    d T_4.

128. The single best predictor of long-term outcome following surgery for gallbladder cancer is:
    a   Positive resection margin.
    b   Nodal status.
    c   Sex of the patient.
    d   Involvement of contiguous organs.

129. The contraindications for surgical therapy in patients with gallbladder cancer include all of the following, except:
    a   Peritoneal disease.
    b   Contiguous liver involvement.
    c   The presence of celiac lymph nodes.
    d   Involvement of the common hepatic artery.

130. A 45-year-old female underwent laparoscopic cholecystectomy for symptomatic gallstones. The subsequent histology shows gallbladder carcinoma involving the perimuscular connective tissue. This patient should be offered:
    a   No further surgical treatment.
    b   Segment IV b and V resection.
    c   Adjuvant chemoradiotherapy.
    d   Follow-up with regular CT scan.

131. A 45-year-old female underwent laparoscopic cholecystectomy for chronic cholecystitis. Histology of the gallbladder shows the presence of carcinoma in situ. The treatment plan for this patient is:
    a No further surgical treatment is necessary.
    b Segment IV b and V resection.
    c Adjuvant chemotherapy.
    d Follow-up with regular CT scan.

132. Which one of the following statements regarding the prognosis of acute pancreatitis is incorrect?
    a Obese patients have a worse prognosis.
    b Patients with no evidence of organ failure in the first week will subsequently develop significant complications.
    c Worsening organ failure is associated with high mortality.
    d Most patients who develop organ dysfunction have some evidence of organ failure at the time of admission.

133. The viral aetiology of acute pancreatitis is suggested by the presence of which one of the following symptoms:
    a Prodromal diarrhoea.
    b Severe epigastric pain radiating to the back.
    c Vomiting.
    d Constipation.

134. An increased immunoglobulin (Ig) G4/IgG ratio is helpful in the diagnosis of:
    a Autoimmune pancreatitis.
    b Hereditary pancreatitis.
    c Tropical pancreatitis.
    d Idiopathic pancreatitis.

135. All of the following procedures are associated with an increased risk of acute pancreatitis following endoscopic retrograde cholangiopancreatography, except:
    a Needle sphincterotomy.
    b Balloon dilatation of benign biliary strictures.
    c Injection of contrast into the pancreatic duct.
    d Endoscopic retrograde cholangiopancreatography and brush cytology.

136. Which of the following statements regarding the management of patients with acute pancreatitis is not true?
   a In patients with severe acute pancreatitis and jaundice there is a role for endoscopic retrograde cholangiopancreatography and sphincterotomy.
   b All patients with acute pancreatitis should receive prophylactic antibiotics.
   c Enteral feeding is the best route of nutritional supplement.
   d All patients with severe acute pancreatitis should be managed in a high dependency/intensive care unit.

137. The most likely diagnosis in a 50-year-old female patient with a recent history of pancreatitis and a large pseudocyst, presenting with sudden onset severe abdominal pain associated with tachycardia and hypotension is:
   a Gram negative septicaemia.
   b Intraperitoneal rupture.
   c Haemorrhage into the pseudocyst.
   d Intragastric rupture.

138. The treatment of choice in a patient with haemorrhage into the pseudocyst secondary to pseudoaneurysm of the splenic artery is:
   a Ligation of the splenic artery.
   b Angiography and splenic artery embolisation.
   c Splenectomy.
   d Conservative treatment with blood transfusion.

139. The most likely cause of gastric varices in a patient with chronic alcoholic pancreatitis is:
   a Portal hypertension secondary to cirrhosis of the liver.
   b Non-cirrhotic portal fibrosis.
   c Portal vein thrombosis.
   d Splenic vein thrombosis.

140. The most common cause of chronic pancreatitis is:
   a Gallstones.
   b Idiopathic.
   c Alcohol.
   d Tropical.

141. The complications associated with chronic pancreatitis include all of the following, except:
   a Cholangiocarcinoma.
   b Gastric outlet obstruction.
   c Obstructive jaundice.
   d Splenic vein thrombosis.

142. The indications for pylorus-preserving pancreaticoduodenectomy in patients with chronic pancreatitis include all of the following, except:
   a Patients with an inflammatory mass in the head of the pancreas.
   b Patients with a large stone in the pancreatic duct associated with pancreatic ductal dilatation.
   c Patients with an inflammatory mass in the head of the pancreas and/causing biliary and duodenal obstruction.
   d Presence of features suggestive of underlying malignancy.

143. The most common type of pancreatic cancer is:
   a Acinar cell carcinoma.
   b Pancreatic ductal carcinoma.
   c Squamous cell carcinoma.
   d Intraductal papillary mucinous neoplasm.

144. All of the following are precursor lesions of pancreatic adenocarcinoma, except:
   a Mucinous cystic neoplasm.
   b Intraductal papillary mucinous neoplasm.
   c Pancreatic intra-epithelial neoplasm.
   d Serous cystadenocarcinoma.

145. In what percentage of patients with painless obstructive jaundice is the gallbladder palpable?
   a >50%.
   b >75%.
   c <25%.
   d In almost all patients.

146. CA 19–9 can be elevated in all of the following conditions, except:
   a Jaundice.
   b Neuroendocrine tumours of the pancreas.
   c Pancreatitis.
   d Pancreatic adenocarcinoma.

147. A 55-year-old male presents with painless obstructive jaundice. Abdominal examination is unremarkable. His alkaline phosphatase (ALP) is 708 U/L, bilirubin 250 μmol/L. Ultrasound scan shows a common bile duct of 10 mm and pancreatic duct of 5 mm diameter. The most likely diagnosis is:

   a Distal common bile duct cholangiocarcinoma.

   b Ampullary carcinoma.

   c Duodenal carcinoma.

   d Carcinoma of the body of the pancreas.

148. The initial diagnostic investigation of choice in patients with obstructive jaundice is:

   a Ultrasound.

   b Endoscopic ultrasound (EUS).

   c Magnetic resonance cholangiopancreatography (MRCP).

   d CT scan.

149. The investigation of choice in the diagnosis and staging of pancreatic cancer is:

   a Magnetic resonance cholangiopancreatography (MRCP).

   b Endoscopic ultrasound (EUS).

   c Triple phase CT.

   d Non-contrast CT.

150. Which one of the following features does not indicate high risk of malignancy in patients with suspected intraductal papillary mucinous neoplasm (IPMN)?

   a Pancreatic duct diameter of >1 cm.

   b Tumour size >3 cm.

   c Presence of mural nodules.

   d Presence of mucin at the ampulla on endoscopic retrograde cholangiopancreatography.

151. The most common site of intraductal papillary mucinous neoplasm (IPMN) is:

   a Ampulla.

   b Head of the pancreas.

   c Body of the pancreas.

   d Tail of the pancreas.

152. The hormone that is commonly elevated in pancreatic neuroendocrine tumours is:
  a 5-hydroxyindoleacetic acid (HIAA).
  b Gastrin.
  c C-peptide.
  d Chromogranin.

153. The most common site of gastrinoma is:
  a Third part of the duodenum.
  b Body of the pancreas.
  c Stomach.
  d Second part of the duodenum.

154. Which of the following statements regarding somatostatin scintigraphy is incorrect?
  a It provides functional images.
  b It is the most sensitive test for the diagnosis of pancreatic neuroendocrine tumours.
  c It provides a detailed anatomical analysis of neuroendocrine tumours.
  d It helps in deciding further treatment with somatostatin analogues.

155. The majority of insulinomas are:
  a Benign.
  b Malignant.
  c More than 2 cm in diameter.
  d Multiple.

156. A 75-year-old male patient with bronchial asthma underwent CT of the chest and abdomen for further evaluation of recent onset cough. It showed a 2 cm lesion in the body of the pancreas. Subsequent endoscopic ultrasound (EUS) and biopsy of the lesion shows features suggestive of a serous cystadenoma. The further management of this patient is:
  a No further treatment required.
  b Distal pancreatectomy.
  c Regular follow-up with CT scan.
  d Enucleation.

157. The most commonly injured solid organ following blunt abdomen injury is the:
   a Liver.
   b Spleen.
   c Kidney.
   d Pancreas.

158. A 25-year-old male is brought to A&E by ambulance crew after being involved in a road traffic incident. On arrival he is conscious, oriented with a GCS of 15/15. He is complaining of severe right lower chest pain. His pulse rate is 100/min and BP 90/60 mmHg. Clinical examination reveals tenderness over the right lower chest. Urgent chest X-ray reveals fractures of the right 7th, 8th and 9th ribs. The initial management of this patient is:
   a Fluid resuscitation.
   b Urgent CT scan.
   c Diagnostic peritoneal lavage (DPL).
   d Laparotomy.

159. The most frequently injured part of the biliary tree following blunt abdominal trauma is the:
   a Gallbladder.
   b Insertion of the cystic duct into the bile duct.
   c Common bile duct.
   d Porta hepatis.

160. A 45-year-old male travelling on a bicycle fell off after hitting a tree. He is brought to A&E and at the time of arrival he is complaining of severe epigastric pain. His observations were normal and stable. On abdominal examination there is tenderness in the epigastric region but is otherwise normal. All his blood tests were normal except serum amylase which is 1,500 IU/L. Subsequent CT abdomen shows peripancreatic oedema and fluid in the lesser sac. The most likely diagnosis is:
   a Traumatic pancreatitis.
   b Transection of the pancreas at the neck.
   c Avulsion of the duodenum at the duodenojejunal flexure.
   d Extrahepatic bile duct injury.

161. The preferred treatment for a patient with traumatic main pancreatic ductal disruption at the neck of the pancreas is:
    a Laparotomy and drainage.
    b Distal pancreatectomy.
    c Pancreaticoduodenostomy.
    d Endoscopic retrograde cholangiopancreatography and stenting.

162. A 30-year-old male patient presents with generalised peritonitis following blunt abdominal trauma. At laparotomy there is free bile in the peritoneal cavity. On further exploration, the extrahepatic bile duct is disrupted approximately 2 cm above the first part of the duodenum. There is no other intra-abdominal injury. The bile duct should be repaired with:
    a End-to-end anastomosis over a T-tube.
    b Roux-en-Y hepaticojejunostomy.
    c Refashioning of the edges and end-to-end anastomosis.
    d Refashioning of the edges and end-to-end anastomosis with a T-tube brought through the normal part of the bile duct.

163. The levels of which one of the following proliferative markers is used in the classification of pancreatic neuroendocrine tumours:
    a Ki-67.
    b PCNA.
    c S-phase fraction.
    d VEGF.

164. The following insulin to glucose ratio is consistent with the diagnosis of insulinoma:
    a >0.4.
    b >0.2.
    c >0.6.
    d >0.1.

165. The following drug is used in the medical treatment of insulinoma:
    a Diazoxide.
    b Metformin.
    c Ranitidine.
    d Minoxidil.

166. Which one of the following statements regarding insulinoma is incorrect?
    a Most of the insulinomas are benign and solitary.
    b The most common site is the head of the pancreas.
    c Surgery is the best treatment option.
    d 95% of insulinomas can be localised through surgical exploration and intra-operative ultrasound.

167. The most common functioning malignant endocrine tumour is:
    a Insulinoma.
    b Somatostatin.
    c Gastrinoma.
    d Glucagonoma.

168. The most common pancreatic endocrine tumour associated with MEN-I syndrome is:
    a Insulinoma.
    b Gastrinoma.
    c Nesidioblastosis.
    d Glucagonoma.

169. The majority of neuroendocrine tumours of the pancreas are:
    a Non-functioning tumours.
    b Insulinomas.
    c Gastrinomas.
    d Somatostatinomas.

170. The most common cystic tumour of the pancreas is:
    a Serous cystadenoma.
    b Intraductal papillary mucinous neoplasm.
    c Mucinous cystadenoma.
    d Serous cystadenocarcinoma.

171. A 65-year-old male recently diagnosed with diabetes presents with upper abdominal pain for the last 3 weeks. Abdominal examination is unremarkable. All biochemical and haematological tests were normal. CT scan of the abdomen shows dilation of the main pancreatic duct with a 2 cm lesion in the head of the pancreas, connected to the main pancreatic duct. Endoscopic retrograde cholangiopancreatography (ERCP) shows patulous ampulla with mucin secretion. The most probable diagnosis is:
   a Serous cystadenoma.
   b Intraductal papillary mucinous neoplasm.
   c Mucinous cystadenoma.
   d Mucinous cystadenocarcinoma.

172. Which one of the following cancers is associated with a best prognosis?
   a Ductal carcinoma of the pancreas.
   b Distal cholangiocarcinoma.
   c Ampullary carcinoma.
   d Duodenal carcinoma.

173. The most common histological type of gallbladder cancer is:
   a Adenocarcinoma.
   b Squamous cell carcinoma.
   c Adenosquamous carcinoma.
   d Small cell carcinoma.

174. Which one of the following conditions is associated with a high risk of gallbladder malignancy?
   a Porcelain gallbladder.
   b Inflammatory bowel disease.
   c Familial adenomatous polyposis.
   d Anomalous junction of the pancreatic biliary duct.

175. A 45-year-old female patient with recurrent epigastric pain is found on ultrasound of the abdomen to have a 1 cm non-mobile lesion suggestive of a polyp. A subsequent CT scan confirmed a 1 cm lesion with no signs of malignancy. This patient should be offered:
a Laparoscopic cholecystectomy.
b Open cholecystectomy.
c 6-monthly ultrasound of the abdomen.
d Reassurance.

176. The further treatment of choice in a 58-year-old female with a type 1b adenocarcinoma of the gallbladder diagnosed following laparoscopic cholecystectomy is:
a No further treatment.
b Segment IV b and V resection along with lymph node clearance.
c Radiotherapy.
d Chemotherapy.

177. The major constituent of bile is:
a Cholesterol.
b Water.
c Bile salts.
d Bile pigments.

178. The concentration of which one of the following substances is twice the normal plasma level in pancreatic secretions?
a Sodium.
b Potassium.
c Bicarbonate.
d Chloride.

179. Secretin stimulates pancreatic secretion rich in:
a Bicarbonate and water.
b Protein digestive enzymes.
c Lipid digestive enzymes.
d Carbohydrate digestive enzymes.

180. Cholecystokinin stimulates pancreatic secretion rich in:
a Water.
b Bicarbonate.
c Digestive enzymes.
d All of the above.

181. Which of the following infections increases the risk of hepatocellular carcinoma (HCC)?
    a   Hepatitis C virus (HCV).
    b   Hepatitis B virus (HBV).
    c   Combined HCV and HBV.
    d   Combined HBV and Hepatitis D virus (HDV).

182. Which of the following statements regarding the risk of hepatocellular carcinoma (HCC) in patients with hepatitis C infection is incorrect?
    a   HCV is the most common risk factor for HCC in Asia.
    b   The annual risk of HCC is 1–4%.
    c   It is not mandatory to have established cirrhosis to develop HCC.
    d   The risk of HCC significantly reduces in patients who respond to antiviral treatment.

183. On Doppler study of the liver, which of the following patterns of blood flow indicates hepatic arterial flow?
    a   Continuous flow.
    b   Pulsatile pattern with reverse flow in systole.
    c   Pulsatile pattern with forward flow.
    d   Continuous flow with changes during the respiratory movement.

184. A high level of which one of the following tumour markers from pancreatic cyst aspirate predicts that the lesion is most likely to be a mucinous cystadenoma?
    a   Carcinoembryonic antigen (CEA).
    b   CA 19–9.
    c   Amylase.
    d   CA-125.

185. Which of the following is not a risk factor for carcinoma of the gallbladder?
    a   Typhoid carriers.
    b   Adenomatous gallbladder polyps.
    c   Choledochal cysts.
    d   Oral contraceptives.

186. The contraindications for medical treatment of gallstones include all of the following, except:
   a Stones less than 15 mm in size.
   b Radio-opaque stones.
   c Calcium bilirubinate and oxalate stones.
   d Non-functioning gallbladder.

187. Bile ductopenia is seen in:
   a Graft versus host disease.
   b Alcoholic hepatitis.
   c Autoimmune hepatitis.
   d Cirrhosis.

188. Which of the following statements regarding fibrolamellar carcinoma of the liver is incorrect?
   a It is more common in females.
   b It tends to occur in younger individuals.
   c It has a better prognosis than hepatocellular carcinoma.
   d In affected patients, serum AFP levels are usually >1,000 µg/L.

189. The most abundant bile acid in the bile is:
   a Chenodeoxycholic acid.
   b Cholic acid.
   c Lithocholic acid.
   d Deoxycholic acid.

190. The functions of bile acid include:
   a Facilitation of excretion of cholesterol in stool.
   b Emulsification of intestinal dietary proteins.
   c Facilitation of intestinal absorption of water soluble vitamins.
   d All of the above.

191. Bile acids are actively re-absorbed in which part of the gastrointestinal tract?
   a Sigmoid colon.
   b Jejunum.
   c Terminal ileum.
   d Transverse colon.

192. Which of the following statements regarding biliary sludge is incorrect?
    a It is composed of cholesterol monohydrate crystals, lecithin-cholesterol crystals, and calcium bilirubinate.
    b It can cause biliary colic, cholecystitis and pancreatitis.
    c Prolonged fasting is a predisposing factor.
    d It does not resolve after stopping total parenteral nutrition.

193. The risk factors for gallstone formation include all of the following, except:
    a Pregnancy.
    b Diabetes.
    c Total parenteral nutrition.
    d Rapid weight loss.

194. Which one of the following antibiotics is associated with the formation of gallstones?
    a Ceftriaxone.
    b Cefuroxime.
    c Cephalexin.
    d Cefoperazone.

195. The most common symptom of primary biliary cirrhosis is:
    a Pruritis.
    b Abdominal pain.
    c Jaundice.
    d Bleeding.

196. The triad of haemobilia includes all of the following clinical signs, except:
    a Pain.
    b Fever.
    c Gastrointestinal bleeding.
    d Jaundice.

197. Which of the following is the preferred treatment modality for annular pancreas causing duodenal obstruction?
    a Whipple's operation.
    b Duodenojejunostomy.
    c Gastrojejunostomy.
    d Jejunocystostomy.

198. The most common complication of pancreatic pseudocysts is:
    a   Rupture.
    b   Infection.
    c   Pressure on the viscera.
    d   Haemorrhage.

199. All of the following are characteristics of idiopathic thrombocyto-
     penic purpura (ITP), except:
    a   Female predominance.
    b   Petechiae, ecchymosis and bleeding.
    c   Splenomegaly.
    d   Increased megakaryocytes in the bone marrow.

200. Spontaneous rupture of the spleen occurs most commonly in
     patients with:
    a   Chronic myeloid leukaemia.
    b   Hereditary spherocytosis.
    c   Infectious mononucleosis.
    d   Typhoid.

201. The most common site of an accessory spleen is:
    a   Lienorenal ligament.
    b   Splenic hilum.
    c   Gastro-splenic ligament.
    d   Greater omentum.

202. Which one of the following characteristics is seen in the peripheral
     blood smear of a patient who underwent splenectomy a long time
     ago?
    a   Döhle bodies.
    b   Hypersegmented neutrophils.
    c   Spherocytes.
    d   Howell-Jolly bodies.

203. Which of the following laboratory determinants is abnormally pro-
     longed in idiopathic thrombocytopenic purpura (ITP)?
    a   Activated partial thromboplastin time (APTT).
    b   Prothrombin time.
    c   Bleeding time.
    d   Clotting time.

204. Splenectomy is most useful in the treatment of:
  a Thrombotic thrombocytopenia.
  b Hereditary spherocytosis.
  c Henoch–Schönlein (HS) purpura.
  d Sickle cell anaemia.

205. Splenectomy is associated with a rapid increase in the count of:
  a Lymphocytes.
  b Monocytes.
  c Platelets.
  d Neutrophils.

Answers: Hepatobiliary and pancreatic surgery

1. d Hepatic artery, hepatic vein and biliary anatomy.

2. b The hepatic artery and bile duct anatomy is regular and identical.

3. a 4 sectors and 9 segments.

4. b It goes through the inferior vena cava and gallbladder.

5. b The ratio between the right and left liver is 60:40.

6. c The central part of the liver lobule has a better supply of oxygen and nutrients.

7. b It receives its arterial supply from both the right and left hepatic arteries.

8. d All of the above.

9. a A remnant of the ductus venosus.

10. b It begins in the plane between segments 2 and 3.

11. d All of the above.

12. b Portal vein.

13. c In 25% of patients part or all of the liver is supplied by a replaced artery.

14. a Absence of the right portal vein.

15. a Right side of the common hepatic duct, liver and cystic duct.

16. d Cystic duct.

17. d a and c.

18. a 10 and 12 o'clock.

19. d Right adrenal gland.

20. a Haemangioma.

21. c There is usually a normal plane between the haemangioma and liver tissue.

22. c Magnetic resonance imaging of the liver.

23. a Symptomatic lesion.

24. d Tyrosinaemia

25. c It is associated with an increased risk of haemorrhage during pregnancy.

26. a Surgery should be considered in all patients.

27. d A benign liver lesion.

28. c It should be resected only if there is a diagnostic uncertainty.

29. a *Escherichia coli, Klebsiella, Bacteroides.*

30. a Cholangitis.

31. b Percutaneous drainage of the liver abscess and interval cholecystectomy.

32. b Amoebic liver abscess.

33. a Dogs.

34. a Pre-malignant tumour.

35. a Surgical excision in all patients.

36. c It can develop in patients with hepatitis E infection.

37. b Oral contraceptive usage.

38. d HBsAg antibody positive patients.

39. a Vaccination against hepatitis B virus.

40. e All of the above.

41. b HCV related HCC is very rare before the age of 40 in the absence of other co-factors.

42. b Tay-Sachs disease.

43. a Gender.

44. d Lungs.

45. a Ruptured hepatocellular carcinoma (HCC).

46. c AFP has low sensitivity and specificity.

47. b Early uptake and early washout.

48. c Magnetic resonance imaging of the liver.

49. a When the mortality from the disease is very high.

50. b Liver resection.

51. b Liver transplantation.

52. a 5 cm suspicious nodule in a cirrhotic liver.

53. a Presence of capsular invasion.

54. a It receives blood supply from the hepatic artery.

55. b Gallstones.

56. e All of the above.

57. b It is more common in females.

58. b Hypovascular.

59. d Neoadjuvant chemotherapy followed by liver and colonic resection.

60. c Unresectable extrahepatic lymph nodal disease.

61. a IgG4.

62. a Steroids.

63. a It is associated with abnormal liver enzymes.

64. b Relaxation of the pylorus.

65. a Manometry.

66. a Usually requires manometry to establish the diagnosis.

67. a Normal pancreatic enzymes.

68. b It acts by inhibiting thymidine phosphorylase.

69. b Right radical nephrectomy and right hemihepatectomy.

70. c Hand-foot syndrome.

71. a Aetiology of the cirrhosis.

72. b Bilirubin, albumin, prothrombin time, ascites and encephalopathy.

73. c Presence of ascites.

74. c 30–40%.

75. b INR, bilirubin and creatinine.

76. a Schistosomiasis.

77. d 9.

78. b 12 mmHg.

79. d Variceal band ligation.

80. b Endoscopic band ligation.

81. a Endoscopic sclerotherapy with cyanoacrylate.

82. b Patients with a prior history of encephalopathy.

83. d Liver transplantation.

84. a Occlusion of the hepatic veins.

85. d Oesophageal variceal haemorrhage.

86. a Clinical tolerance.

87. a Transjugular intrahepatic portosystemic shunt (TIPS).

88. d Splenectomy.

89. a Pneumococcal, *H influenzae*, meningococcal.

90. a *Streptococcus pneumoniae*.

91. c Fluid resuscitation.

92. a Grade 1 and 2 injury.

93. a Mixed cholesterol and pigment stones.

94. b Repeat ultrasound scan.

95. a Haemolytic anaemia.

96. b Loss of equilibrium between phospholipids, cholesterol and bile salts.

97. b Endoscopic ultrasound (EUS).

98. a Cholesterol metabolism.

99. d Endoscopic retrograde cholangiopancreatography and stone extraction.

100. c Reassurance.

101. b She should be considered for laparoscopic banding and cholecystectomy at the same time.

102. b Hepatobiliary scintigraphy.

103. d Acute cholecystitis.

104. b Complete excision of the cyst followed by Roux-en-Y hepaticojejunostomy.

105. b Pancreatic carcinoma.

106. c Bile leak.

107. b Consider repeat laparoscopy and washout.

108. a Cystic duct stump leak.

109. b Early repair of the bile duct by a hepatobiliary and pancreatic surgeon.

110. d All of the above.

111. d Gallbladder.

112. a Hilum.

113. d Gallstones.

114. d Chronic pancreatitis.

115. d Papillary type is associated with a good prognosis.

116. d It is essential to make a histological diagnosis before treatment.

117. c Carcinoma of the head of the pancreas.

118. e a and d.

119. b Risk of cholangitis.

120. c Tumour involving the biliary confluence.

121. d Caudate lobe resection is not associated with improved negative margins.

122. c Poorly-differentiated histology.

123. a Percutaneous drainage of the left ductal system.

124. d Previous endoscopic sphincterotomy.

125. c Patients with asymptomatic gallstones.

126. a Patients with cirrhosis.

127. d T_4.

128. b Nodal status.

129. b Contiguous liver involvement.

130. b Segment IV b and V resection.

131. a No further surgical treatment is necessary.

132. b Patients with no evidence of organ failure in the first week will subsequently develop significant complications.

133. a Prodromal diarrhoea.

134. a Autoimmune pancreatitis.

135. d Endoscopic retrograde cholangiopancreatography and brush cytology.

136.   b   All patients with acute pancreatitis should receive prophylactic antibiotics.

137.   c   Haemorrhage into the pseudocyst.

138.   b   Angiography and splenic artery embolisation.

139.   d   Splenic vein thrombosis.

140.   c   Alcohol.

141.   a   Cholangiocarcinoma.

142.   b   Patients with a large stone in the pancreatic duct associated with pancreatic ductal dilatation.

143.   b   Pancreatic ductal carcinoma.

144.   d   Serous cystadenocarcinoma.

145.   c   <25%.

146.   b   Neuroendocrine tumours of the pancreas.

147.   b   Ampullary carcinoma.

148.   a   Ultrasound.

149.   c   Triple phase CT.

150.   d   Presence of mucin at the ampulla on endoscopic retrograde cholangiopancreatography.

151.   b   Head of the pancreas.

152.   d   Chromogranin.

153.   d   Second part of the duodenum.

154.   c   It provides a detailed anatomical analysis of neuroendocrine tumours.

155. a Benign.

156. c Regular follow-up with CT scan.

157. b Spleen.

158. a Fluid resuscitation.

159. a Gallbladder.

160. a Traumatic pancreatitis.

161. d Endoscopic retrograde cholangiopancreatography and stenting.

162. b Roux-en-Y hepaticojejunostomy.

163. a Ki-67.

164. a >0.4.

165. a Diazoxide.

166. b The most common site is the head of the pancreas.

167. c Gastrinoma.

168. b Gastrinoma.

169. a Non-functioning tumours.

170. c Mucinous cystadenoma.

171. b Intraductal papillary mucinous neoplasm.

172. c Ampullary carcinoma.

173. a Adenocarcinoma.

174. a Porcelain gallbladder.

175. a Laparoscopic cholecystectomy.

176. b Segment IV b and V resection along with lymph node clearance.

177. b Water.

178. c Bicarbonate.

179. a Bicarbonate and water.

180. d All of the above.

181. c Combined HCV and HBV.

182. c It is not mandatory to have established cirrhosis to develop HCC.

183. c Pulsatile pattern with forward flow.

184. a Carcinoembryonic antigen (CEA).

185. d Oral contraceptives.

186. a Stones less than 15 mm in size.

187. a Graft versus host disease.

188. d In affected patients, serum AFP levels are usually >1,000 µg/L.

189. a Chenodeoxycholic acid.

190. a Facilitation of excretion of cholesterol in stool.

191. c Terminal ileum.

192. d It does not resolve after stopping total parenteral nutrition.

193. b Diabetes.

194. a Ceftriaxone.

195. a Pruritis.

196. b Fever.

197. b Duodenojejunostomy.

198. b Infection.

199. c Splenomegaly.

200. c Infectious mononucleosis.

201. b Splenic hilum.

202. d Howell-Jolly bodies.

203. c Bleeding time.

204. b Hereditary spherocytosis.

205. c Platelets.

5
Transplantation

Questions

1. One of the following is not a contraindication for cadaveric kidney donation:
   a Age >65 years.
   b Longstanding hypertension.
   c Diabetes.
   d Intra-abdominal malignancy.

2. All of the following are absolute contraindications for organ donation, except:
   a Untreated systemic sepsis.
   b Hepatic malignancy.
   c HIV infection.
   d Intracranial malignancy.

3. All of the following except one criterion is used to establish brain stem death in the UK:
   a Fixed and dilated pupil not responding to light.
   b Absent EEG activity.
   c Absent corneal reflexes.
   d No occulocephalic reflex.

4. Before establishing brain stem death, the following criteria should be satisfied:
   a Reversible causes for brain stem dysfunction should be excluded.
   b Drugs liable to cause depression of conscious level should be excluded.
   c Patient must not have received neuromuscular blocking drugs in the past.
   d All reversible causes should be excluded.
   e All of the above.

5. All of the following except one is a contraindication for organ donation:
   a Active sepsis.
   b Colon cancer.
   c Basal cell carcinoma.
   d High-grade melanoma.

6. All of the following hormonal changes are associated with brain stem death, except:
   a Hyperthyroidism.
   b Diabetes insipidus.
   c Diabetes mellitus.
   d Hypothermia.

7. The rationale behind using impermeable substrates (impermeants) in organ preservation solution is:
   a They counteract cellular swelling by adding osmotic force.
   b They prevent high intracellular potassium and calcium.
   c They lower the metabolic activity of the cell.
   d None of the above.

8. The impermeant used in hyperosmolar citrate solution is:
   a Citrate.
   b Glucose.
   c Mannitol.
   d Raffinose.

9. All of the following except one is a constituent of University of Wisconsin solution:
   a Raffinose and lactobionate.
   b Sodium bicarbonate.
   c Potassium chloride.
   d Glucose.

10. The best preservation solution for a kidney is:
    a University of Wisconsin.
    b Euro-Collins solution.
    c Hyperosmolar citrate.
    d Phosphate buffer sucrose.

11. The rationale behind the administration of methylprednisolone before organ retrieval is:
    a It prevents release of lytic enzymes by stabilising the lysozomes.
    b It lowers the metabolic activity of the cell.
    c It acts as an antioxidant.
    d It reduces interstitial space expansion.

12. Which one of the following is not a constituent of Marshall's solution?
    a Potassium phosphate.
    b Mannitol.
    c Sodium citrate.
    d Potassium citrate.

13. Allograft is:
    a Transplantation of an organ within an animal.
    b Transplantation between genetically identical twins.
    c Transplantation between non-genetically identical members of the same species.
    d Transplantation between genetically identical members of different species.

14. Which one of the following statements regarding hyperacute rejection is incorrect?
    a It is a cell mediated phenomenon.
    b It can be due to previous blood transfusion.
    c It results in graft destruction within a few hours of transplantation.
    d It may occur due to naturally occurring antibodies.

15. Acute rejection most commonly occurs:
    a Within a few hours of transplantation.
    b Between day 5 and 14 following transplantation.
    c 1 to 3 days following transplantation.
    d Any time after 3 months of transplantation.

16. Encoding for the major histocompatibility complex (MHC) antigens is present on which of the following chromosomes:
    a Short arm of chromosome 6.
    b Short arm of chromosome 11.
    c Short arm of chromosome 17.
    d Short arm of chromosome 5.

17. Class I major histocompatibility complex (MHC) antigens are present in almost all nucleated cells, except:
    a Red blood cell.
    b Corneal endothelial cell.
    c Platelets.
    d T-lymphocyte.

18. Hepatic artery thrombosis can be associated with:
    a Mycophenolate mofetil.
    b Tacrolimus.
    c Steroids.
    d Rapamycin.

19. Gingival hyperplasia is a side-effect of:
    a Ciclosporin.
    b Tacrolimus.
    c Mycophenolate mofetil.
    d Sirolimus.

20. All of the following are side-effects associated with ciclosporin, except:
    a Hepatic artery thrombosis.
    b Gingival hyperplasia.
    c Hypertension.
    d Hypertrichosis.

21. The following immunosuppressive agent is an anti-metabolite:
    a Ciclosporin.
    b Tacrolimus
    c Mycophenolate.
    d Rapamycin.

22. The mechanism of action of sirolimus is:
    a It inhibits calcineurin activity.
    b It inhibits the mammalian target of rapamycin.
    c It is a monoclonal antibody of IL-2 receptor.
    d It inhibits the conversion of IMP to GMP.

23. The immunosuppressive agent OKT-3 acts by:
   a Inhibiting interleukin-2 receptor α.
   b It is an anti-CD 25 monoclonal antibody.
   c It is an anti-CD 3 monoclonal antibody.
   d It is an anti-CD 4 monoclonal antibody.

24. Cytokine release syndrome is a side-effect of which one of the following immunosuppressive agents?
   a Azathioprine.
   b Tacrolimus.
   c Sirolimus.
   d OKT-3.

25. The mechanism of action of Basiliximab is:
   a It is an IL-2 receptor monoclonal antibody.
   b It is an anti-CD 3 monoclonal antibody.
   c It is a calcineurin inhibitor.
   d It is an anti-CD 25 monoclonal antibody.

26. Which one of the following immunosuppressive agents is a monoclonal antibody to CD 25?
   a Basiliximab.
   b OKT-3.
   c Daclizumab.
   d Rapamycin.

27. The main side-effect of ciclosporin is:
   a Neurotoxicity.
   b Nephrotoxicity.
   c Hypokalaemia.
   d Hypoglycaemia.

28. Which one of the following statements regarding tacrolimus is incorrect?
   a Its absorption is not influenced by bile.
   b Food reduces its bio-availability.
   c It is more potent than ciclosporin.
   d Antifungal agents reduce its blood levels.

29. Which of the following prokinetic agents can affect the blood tacrolimus levels?
a Metoclopramide.
b Erythromycin.
c Domperidone.
d a and b.

30. Diarrhoea is the side-effect of which of the following immunosuppressive agents?
a Mycophenolate mofetil.
b Azathioprine.
c Tacrolimus.
d Ciclosporin.

31. Myelosuppression is the side-effect of which of the following immunosuppressive agents?
a Tacrolimus.
b Azathioprine.
c Corticosteroid.
d Ciclosporin.

32. Which one of the following immunosuppressive agents augments the bio-availability of mycophenolate mofetil?
a Tacrolimus.
b Azathioprine.
c Corticosteroid.
d Rapamycin.

33. Which one of the following immunosuppressive agents has anti-tumour and anti-fungal properties?
a Tacrolimus.
b Azathioprine.
c Corticosteroid.
d Sirolimus.

34. All of the following are side-effects of tacrolimus, except:
a Renal dysfunction.
b Hypertension.
c Hyperkalaemia.
d Diabetes insipidus.

35. Inosine monophosphate dehydrogenase is a critical rate limiting enzyme in the so-called de novo synthesis of purines and catalyses the formation of guanosine nucleotides from inosine. Which one of the following immunosuppressive drugs works by inhibiting this enzyme?
    a Mycophenolate mofetil.
    b Azathioprine.
    c Tacrolimus.
    d Sirolimus.

36. All of the following are contraindications for living related kidney donation, except:
    a Single episode of nephrolithiasis.
    b Diabetes.
    c Hypertension.
    d Family history of renal cell carcinoma.

37. Which one of the following is not a contraindication for living kidney donation?
    a Obesity (BMI >35).
    b Active alcohol abuse.
    c Collagen vascular disease.
    d Cervical cancer in situ.

38. The contraindications for cadaveric kidney donation include:
    a Chronic renal disease.
    b Severe hypertension.
    c Hepatitis B surface antigen positive.
    d All of the above.

39. Which one of the following statements regarding donors from cardiac death compared to donors from brain stem death is incorrect?
    a It is associated with an increased risk of delayed graft function.
    b It is associated with worse overall graft survival.
    c It is associated with an increased risk of primary graft dysfunction.
    d Serum creatinine at 2 and 5 years is higher.

40. The electrolyte abnormalities associated with early post-renal transplantation are:
   a Hyperkalaemia, hypernatraemia, hypomagnesaemia, hypophosphataemia.
   b Hypokalaemia, hyponatraemia, hypermagnesaemia, hypophosphataemia.
   c Hypokalaemia, hyponatraemia, hypomagnesaemia, hypophosphataemia.
   d Hyperphosphataemia, hypernatraemia, hypokalaemia, hyperphosphataemia.

41. The electrolyte abnormalities associated with bladder drained pancreatic transplantation are:
   a Hyponatraemia, metabolic acidosis.
   b Hyponatraemia, hypokalaemia, metabolic alkalosis.
   c Hypernatraemia, hyperkalaemia, metabolic acidosis.
   d Hyponatraemia, hyperkalaemia, metabolic alkalosis.

42. The initial warm ischaemia time during donation from brain stem death donors is defined as:
   a The time interval between aortic clamping until perfusion with cold preservation fluid.
   b Time interval between circulatory arrest and commencement of perfusion with cold preservation fluid.
   c The time interval from removal of the organ from cold storage until vascularisation of the graft.
   d The time interval between removal of the organ from the body until it is stored in cold storage fluid.

43. Prolonged warm ischaemia time is associated with:
   a Increased delayed graft function.
   b Increased primary graft failure.
   c Increased chronic rejection.
   d a and b.

44. The most common cause of sudden death following living related kidney donation is:
   a Myocardial infarction.
   b Pulmonary embolism.
   c Air embolism.
   d Tension pneumothorax.

45. The following criterion is used in the selection of recipient for reduced size graft:
   a Ratio based on the donor to recipient weight.
   b Ratio based on the donor to recipient age.
   c Ratio based on the donor to recipient body mass index (BMI).
   d Ratio based on the donor to recipient height.

46. Reduction in the size of liver graft is necessary if the donor/recipient weight ratio is:
   a 2 or more.
   b 5 or less.
   c 5 or more.
   d 10 or more.

47. A 45-year-old male patient presents to A&E 2 weeks following liver transplantation with diarrhoea for the last 3 days. On examination he is pyrexial with a temperature of 38°C, pulse rate 110/min, with normal blood pressure. His liver function test shows AST of 2,100 IU/L and his ALP is 110 IU/L at the time of discharge. What is the most likely diagnosis?
   a Acute rejection.
   b Hepatic artery thrombosis.
   c Cytomegalovirus infection.
   d Diarrhoea related to immunosuppressive agents.

48. Compared to whole liver transplantation, split liver transplant is associated with an increased risk of:
   a Hepatic artery thrombosis.
   b Primary non-function.
   c Delayed graft function.
   d Poor overall survival.

49. A 50-year-old male patient with A+ blood group received a liver transplant from an O+ donor. The donor haemoglobin has dropped to 5 gm/dL 48 hours following transplantation. The recipient should receive:
a A+ blood.
b O+ blood.
c AB+ blood.
d A- blood.

50. The most common hepatic artery anatomical variation is:
a Left hepatic artery from left gastric artery (12%).
b Accessory right hepatic artery from superior mesenteric artery.
c Replaced right hepatic artery from superior mesenteric artery.
d Left gastric artery from left hepatic artery (7%).

51. The risk of acute rejection following orthoptic liver transplantation is highest at:
a 3–6 months.
b <2 months.
c 1–3 months.
d After 12 months.

52. Absolute contraindications for liver transplantation include all, except:
a Extrahepatic organ failure.
b Severe uncontrollable sepsis.
c Colorectal liver metastasis.
d Liver metastases from small bowel carcinoid tumour.

53. For every 10°C drop in temperature the metabolic activity of the donor organ is decreased by:
a 1.5–2 fold.
b 5–10 fold.
c 10–15 fold.
d 15–20 fold.

54. A kidney biopsy from a transplanted kidney 12 months following transplantation shows features of tubular atrophy, interstitial fibrosis and fibro-intimal thickening of the arteries. These changes most likely represent:
    a Changes associated with chronic rejection.
    b Changes associated with ciclosporin nephrotoxicity.
    c Changes associated with mycophenolate-induced nephrotoxicity.
    d Changes associated with diabetic nephropathy.

55. The indications for renal replacement therapy include:
    a Metabolic acidosis.
    b Pulmonary oedema.
    c Plasma urea >30 mmol/L and creatinine >600 μmol/L.
    d All of the above.

56. Complications associated with haemodialysis include all, except:
    a Hypotension.
    b Cardiac arrhythmias.
    c Air embolism.
    d Hyperkalaemia.

57. HLA matching is necessary for the transplantation of the:
    a Kidney.
    b Liver.
    c Lung.

58. The most common reason for not using a donor liver following retrieval is:
    a Severe steatosis.
    b Poor perfusion.
    c Prolonged cold ischaemia time.
    d Damage to donor liver during retrieval.

59. Portacaval shunt during a hepatic phase is associated with all of the following advantages, except:
    a Reduced intra-operative requirements for blood transfusion.
    b Decreased intestinal congestion.
    c Preserved renal function.
    d Poor haemodynamic tolerance.

60. The risk factors that predict recurrence of hepatocellular cancer following liver transplantation include all, except:

   a Tumour sizes of less than 5 cm.
   b Vascular invasion.
   c Lymph node involvement.
   d α-fetoprotein (AFP) of >300 IU/L.

Answers: Transplantation

1. a Age >65 years.

2. d Intracranial malignancy.

3. b Absent EEG activity.

4. e All of the above.

5. c Basal cell carcinoma.

6. a Hyperthyroidism.

7. a They counteract cellular swelling by adding osmotic force.

8. c Mannitol.

9. d Glucose.

10. c Hyperosmolar citrate.

11. a It prevents release of lytic enzymes by stabilising the lysozomes.

12. a Potassium phosphate.

13. c Transplantation between non-genetically identical members of the same species.

14. a It is a cell mediated phenomenon.

15. b Between day 5 and 14 following transplantation.

16. **a** Short arm of chromosome 6.

17. **b** Corneal endothelial cell.

18. **d** Rapamycin.

19. **a** Ciclosporin.

20. **a** Hepatic artery thrombosis.

21. **c** Mycophenolate.

22. **b** It inhibits the mammalian target of rapamycin.

23. **c** It is an anti-CD 3 monoclonal antibody.

24. **d** OKT-3.

25. **a** It is an IL-2 receptor monoclonal antibody.

26. **c** Daclizumab.

27. **b** Nephrotoxicity.

28. **d** Antifungal agents reduce its blood levels.

29. **d** a and b.

30. **a** Mycophenolate mofetil.

31. **b** Azathioprine.

32. **a** Tacrolimus.

33. **d** Sirolimus.

34. **d** Diabetes insipidus.

35. **a** Mycophenolate mofetil.

36. **a** Single episode of nephrolithiasis.

37. **d** Cervical cancer in situ.

38. **d** All of the above.

39. **b** It is associated with worse overall graft survival.

40. **a** Hyperkalaemia, hypernatraemia, hypomagnesaemia, hypophosphataemia.

41. **a** Hyponatraemia, metabolic acidosis.

42. **a** The time interval between aortic clamping until perfusion with cold preservation fluid.

43. **d** a and b.

44. **b** Pulmonary embolism.

45. **a** Ratio based on the donor to recipient weight.

46. **a** 2 or more.

47. **b** Hepatic artery thrombosis.

48. **a** Hepatic artery thrombosis.

49. **b** O+ blood.

50. **a** Left hepatic artery from left gastric artery (12%).

51. **c** 1–3 months.

52. **d** Liver metastases from small bowel carcinoid tumour.

53. **a** 1.5–2 fold.

54. **a** Changes associated with chronic rejection.

55. **d** All of the above.

56. **d** Hyperkalaemia.

57. a Kidney.

58. a Severe steatosis.

59. d Poor haemodynamic tolerance.

60. a Tumour sizes of less than 5 cm.

6

Vascular surgery

Questions

1. Klippel-Trenaunay syndrome (KTS) is a congenital disorder that affects the:
   a Capillaries.
   b Lymphatics.
   c Veins.
   d All of the above.

2. Which of the following is not a component of Klippel-Trenaunay syndrome (KTS)?
   a Varicose veins.
   b Limb length discrepancies.
   c Port wine stains.
   d Muscular atrophy.

3. Which one of the following statements with regard to arteriovenous (AV) malformation is incorrect?
   a AV malformations are direct arteriovenous communications.
   b AV malformations can be associated with congestive heart failure.
   c AV malformations may be associated with swelling and venous engorgement.
   d AV malformations are often clinically inactive in the first and second decade of life.

4. Which of the following is not a side-effect of treatment of venous malformation using sclerosing agents?
   a Deep vein thrombosis.
   b Haemoglobinuria.
   c Pulmonary hypertension.
   d Gastric ulcer.

5. During treatment with a large amount of sclerosing agents for vascular malformation, the following measures are used to prevent acute renal failure associated with haemoglobinuria:
   a Intravenous fluids.
   b Intravenous sodium bicarbonate administration.
   c Intravenous mannitol.
   d All of the above.

6. Which one of the following is not a sclerosing agent?
   a Ethanol.
   b Sodium tetradecyl sulfate.
   c Polidocanol
   d Ethiodol.

7. A 55-year-old female presents with sudden onset severe right calf pain for 24 hours. On clinical examination she has right leg oedema associated with tenderness in the calf. The most likely diagnosis is:
   a Deep vein thrombosis.
   b Ruptured popliteal cyst.
   c Cellulitis.
   d Congestive heart failure.

8. An 18-year-old female presents with a 2-week history of swollen leg following a right ankle sprain. The most likely diagnosis is:
   a Deep vein thrombosis.
   b Ruptured popliteal cyst.
   c Cellulitis.
   d Lymphoedema praecox.

9. A 35-year-old male with obstructive jaundice due to pancreatic carcinoma is admitted for percutaneous transhepatic biliary drainage following failed endoscopic retrograde cholangiopancreaticography (ERCP). 24 hours post-procedure he develops a deep vein thrombosis of his right leg. He should be treated with anticoagulant for a minimum period of:
   a 6 months.
   b 12 months.
   c Until definite surgery.
   d Life-long.

10. A 50-year-old female patient develops deep vein thrombosis (DVT) following total knee replacement. Anticoagulant therapy should be given for a period of:
    a Life-long.
    b 3 months.
    c 6 months.
    d 12 months.

11. The investigation of choice for the diagnosis of deep vein thrombosis is:
    a Plethysmography.
    b Venous duplex scan.
    c Venography.
    d MRI.

12. The most common site of a varicose venous ulcer is:
    a Medial aspect of lower leg.
    b Lateral aspect of lower leg.
    c Heal of the foot.
    d Over the calf.

13. Which of the following clinical features is not a feature of venous claudication?
    a Bursting sensation after exercise.
    b Pain relief immediately after the cessation of exercise.
    c Pain relief after elevation of leg.
    d Generalised pain in leg following exercise.

14. The amount of pressure produced by class II compression stockings used for chronic venous insufficiency is:
    a <25 mmHg.
    b 25–35 mmHg.
    c 35–45 mmHg.
    d 45–60 mmHg.

15. The following class of compression stocking is recommended for the treatment of patients with severe lymphoedema due to chronic venous insufficiency:
    a Class I.
    b Class II.
    c Class III.
    d Class IV.

16. The CEAP classification system is used to describe the severity and aetiology of:
    a Lower limb venous disease.
    b Lower limb arterial disease.
    c Lower limb lymphatic disease.
    d All of the above.

17. Lipodermatosclerosis is associated with:
    a Chronic venous insufficiency.
    b Peripheral arterial disease.
    c Chronic lymphoedema.
    d a and c.

18. The nerve at risk of damage during stripping of the long saphenous vein is the:
    a Sural nerve.
    b Femoral nerve.
    c Superficial peroneal nerve.
    d Saphenous nerve.

19. The nerve at risk of damage during saphenopopliteal disconnection is the:
    a Superficial peroneal nerve.
    b Common peroneal nerve.
    c Sural nerve.
    d Saphenous nerve.

20. The following nerve is at risk of damage during stripping of the short saphenous vein:
    a Sural nerve.
    b Femoral nerve.
    c Superficial peroneal nerve.
    d Saphenous nerve.

21. Endovenous LASER ablation therapy for varicose veins is associated with all of the following advantages, except:
    a Reduced risk of nerve injury.
    b It avoids neovascularisation.
    c It does not treat the varices.
    d It is associated with less morbidity.

22. A 50-year-old male patient presents with severe bleeding following scratching of the skin over a prominent vein on the right medial aspect of the leg. The best option to control the bleeding is:
    a   Pressure application and elevation of the leg.
    b   Apply tourniquet above the bleeding point.
    c   Explore the wound under local anaesthesia and ligate the source of bleeding.
    d   Urgent saphenofemoral junction ligation and stripping.

23. The preferred central vein for venous catheterisation is the:
    a   Subclavian vein.
    b   Cephalic vein.
    c   Internal jugular vein.
    d   Brachial vein.

24. The right internal jugular vein is the preferred site for central venous catheterisation because:
    a   It provides a direct route to the superior vena cava.
    b   It is associated with no complications.
    c   It can be used for a long duration.
    d   There is less risk of damage to the thoracic duct.

25. Arteriovenous fistulas are preferred over arteriovenous grafts for providing access to haemodialysis for all of the following reasons, except:
    a   Lower infection rate.
    b   Higher patency.
    c   Requires fewer revisions.
    d   Can be used as soon as the wounds have healed.

26. Which of the following is the contraindication for varicose vein surgery?
    a   Deep vein thrombosis.
    b   Ankle flare.
    c   Lipodermatosclerosis.
    d   Venous bleeding.

27. The most common cause of arteriovenous fistula graft dysfunction is:
    a   Stenosis.
    b   Infection.
    c   Thrombosis.
    d   Steal phenomenon.

28. The majority of stenosed arteriovenous fistulas can be treated with:
    a Angioplasty.
    b Stenting.
    c Surgical repair.
    d Thrombolysis.

29. How long before the anticipated need for dialysis should arterio-venous fistulas be constructed?
    a <1 week.
    b 1–2 weeks.
    c 2–4 weeks.
    d 4–6 weeks.

30. What percentage of arteriovenous fistulas remains patent but never achieves an adequate flow for dialysis?
    a 1%.
    b 5%.
    c 10%.
    d 25%.

31. The most preferred site for the formation of an arteriovenous fistula is the:
    a Radiocephalic fistula.
    b Ulnabasilic fistula.
    c Brachiocephalic fistula.
    d Brachiobasilic fistula.

32. The most common cause of acute mesenteric ischaemia is:
    a Embolic occlusion of the superior mesenteric artery.
    b Thrombosis of the superior mesenteric artery.
    c Stenosis of the superior mesenteric artery.
    d Iatrogenic occlusion of the superior mesenteric artery with endograft.

33. The artery not affected by Takayasu's arteritis is the:
    a Radial artery.
    b Subclavian artery.
    c Common carotid artery.
    d Renal artery.

34. A 75-year-old female with peripheral arterial disease and angina presents with a 3-month history of post-prandial abdominal pain associated with progressive weight loss. On clinical examination the patient is lean with no other obvious findings. The most likely diagnosis is:
   a Peptic ulcer disease.
   b Chronic mesenteric ischaemia.
   c Diverticular disease.
   d Gastric malignancy.

35. The most common cause of true visceral artery aneurysm is:
   a Trauma.
   b Mycotic.
   c Atherosclerosis.
   d Syphilis.

36. The most common site of visceral artery aneurysm is the:
   a Hepatic artery.
   b Superior mesenteric artery.
   c Celiac artery.
   d Splenic artery.

37. A 65-year-old male patient is diagnosed with a 6.5 cm descending thoracic aneurysm following investigation for non-specific chest pain. Apart from the history of mild angina, the patient is fit and healthy. The treatment of choice is:
   a No treatment required.
   b Open surgical repair.
   c Endovascular repair.
   d Surveillance by computed tomography (CT) scan.

38. The most common complication associated with endovascular repair of a thoracic aortic aneurysm is:
   a Infection.
   b Spinal cord ischaemia.
   c Endoleak.
   d Upper limb ischaemia.

39. All of the following conditions are associated with thoracic aorta aneurysm, except:
  a Marfan's syndrome.
  b Turner syndrome.
  c Reiter's disease.
  d Ehlers-Danlos syndrome.

40. The treatment of choice in a patient with complicated type B thoracic aortic dissection is:
  a Open surgical repair.
  b Endovascular repair.
  c Medical management.
  d None of the above.

41. The most common site of traumatic thoracic aortic injury is:
  a Isthmus of the aorta.
  b Root of the aorta.
  c Lower part of the descending thoracic aorta.
  d Arch of the aorta.

42. Which one of the following statements regarding the prevalence of abdominal aortic aneurysm is incorrect?
  a It is six times more common in women.
  b 25% of patients have co-existing femoral and popliteal artery aneurysms.
  c Prevalence increases with age.
  d Infrarenal aortic aneurysm is the most common abdominal aortic aneurysm.

43. Which one of the following statements regarding infrarenal aortic aneurysm is incorrect?
  a 75% of patients are symptomatic at the time of diagnosis.
  b Rapid expansion of >1 cm is an indication for intervention.
  c 75% of patients with rupture die before reaching the hospital.
  d Infrarenal aortic aneurysm >5.5 cm is an indication for intervention.

44. The investigation of choice used in the screening for abdominal aortic aneurysm is:
  a Doppler ultrasound.
  b Ultrasound.
  c Computed tomography (CT) scan.
  d Magnetic resonance imaging (MRI).

45. The annual risk of rupture of an abdominal aortic aneurysm measuring 4–5 cm is:
   a 0%.
   b 9.4%.
   c 3.3%.
   d 1.1%.

46. In the UK Small Aneurysm Trial the rupture rate for an untreated small aneurysm is:
   a <2%.
   b 2–4%.
   c 0%.
   d 9.4%.

47. The most appropriate interval for screening of abdominal aortic aneurysms between 4.5–5.4 cm is:
   a 3 months.
   b 6 months.
   c 12 months.
   d 24 months.

48. Survival following abdominal aortic aneurysm rupture is poor in all of the following groups of patients, except:
   a Elderly patients.
   b Patients who suffered from cardiac arrest.
   c Patients who are persistently unconscious.
   d Patients with low/absent urine output.

49. Which one of the following factors is not included in the calculation of the Glasgow aneurysm score used in the risk stratification for assessing a patient's suitability for abdominal aortic aneurysm surgery?
   a Age.
   b Size of aneurysm.
   c Renal dysfunction.
   d History of cerebrovascular disease.

50. The size of asymptomatic common iliac aneurysm above which treatment is indicated is:
    a 2.5 cm.
    b 2.5–3 cm.
    c 3–4 cm.
    d >4 cm.

51. The most common site of true peripheral artery aneurysm is:
    a Femoral.
    b Popliteal.
    c Brachial.
    d Radial.

52. Which one of the following statements regarding popliteal artery aneurysm is correct?
    a It is the most common peripheral aneurysm.
    b >75% are bilateral.
    c One-third of them are asymptomatic.
    d 40% are associated with abdominal aortic aneurysm.

53. The preferred treatment in a patient with a popliteal artery aneurysm of less than 2 cm is:
    a Proximal and distal ligation.
    b Proximal and distal ligation and bypass using autologous vein.
    c Proximal and distal ligation and bypass using synthetic graft.
    d An inlay graft repair.

54. A 50-year-old male patient with a previous history of popliteal artery aneurysm on the right side is found to have a 2 cm thrombosed popliteal artery aneurysm on the left side by ultrasound surveillance. The most appropriate treatment is:
    a Proximal and distal ligation.
    b Proximal and distal ligation and bypass using autologous vein.
    c Proximal and distal ligation and bypass using synthetic graft.
    d An inlay graft repair.

55. The most commonly used calcium-channel blocker in the treatment of Raynaud's syndrome is:
    a Nifedipine.
    b Verapamil.
    c Naftidrofuryl oxalate.
    d Ketanserin.

56. Which of the following drugs is associated with Raynaud's phenomenon?
a   Calcium-channel blockers.
b   β-blockers.
c   ACE inhibitors.
d   Erythromycin.

57. The sequence of classical manifestations of Raynaud's phenomenon is:
a   Pallor, cyanosis, rubor.
b   Cyanosis, pallor, rubor.
c   Rubor, cyanosis, pallor.
d   Rubor, pallor, cyanosis.

58. Which of the following statements regarding Takayasu's arteritis is incorrect?
a   It commonly affects men.
b   It usually presents between 10 and 30 years of age.
c   It affects all levels of the aorta.
d   Pulmonary artery involvement is present in 50% of patients.

59. The histological feature that is the hallmark of Buerger's disease is:
a   Vessel wall necrosis.
b   Vascular wall calcification.
c   Atheromatous plaques.
d   Acute hypercellular occlusive thrombus.

60. The most commonly affected arteries in Buerger's disease are the:
a   Small and medium arteries of the distal limb.
b   Medium-sized arteries of the proximal lower limb.
c   Medium-sized arteries of the upper limb.
d   Medium-sized arteries of the neck.

61. The risk factor for Buerger's disease is:
a   Age.
b   Diabetes.
c   Smoking.
d   Family history of Buerger's disease.

62. A 54-year-old female presents with sudden loss of vision in her right eye. She also has a history of intermittent temporal headache associated with fatigue and weight loss for the last 6–9 months. On clinical examination, she is blind in her right eye and there is tenderness over the superficial temporal area. The most likely cause of her symptoms is:
    a Temporal arteritis.
    b Takayasu's arteritis.
    c Carotid artery stenosis.
    d Polyarteritis nodosa.

63. The mainstay of treatment of giant cell arteritis is:
    a Corticosteroids.
    b Methotrexate.
    c Calcium and vitamin D therapy.
    d NSAIDs.

64. Buerger's disease affects the:
    a Tunica intima.
    b Tunica media.
    c Tunica adventitia.
    d All of the above.

65. The neurological symptoms associated with thoracic outlet syndrome are mainly due to compression of:
    a C4, 5 nerve roots.
    b C5, 6 nerve roots.
    c C7, 8 nerve roots.
    d C8, T1 nerve roots.

66. The majority of patients with thoracic outlet syndrome present with:
    a Arterial symptoms.
    b Venous symptoms.
    c Neurological symptoms.
    d Arterial and venous symptoms.

67. The most common cause of ischaemic stroke is:
    a Thromboembolism of the internal carotid artery.
    b Small vessel disease.
    c Cardiogenic brain embolism.
    d Fibromuscular dysplasia of the carotid artery.

68. Which one of the following features is not a classical symptom associated with thromboembolism of the carotid artery?
 a Hemi-motor weakness.
 b Amaurosis fugax.
 c Dysphagia.
 d Homonymous hemianopia.

69. The ABCD scoring system is used to predict the:
 a 7-day risk of stroke after a transient ischaemic attack.
 b Risk of mortality following a transient ischaemic attack.
 c 7-day risk of mortality following a stroke.
 d Response to medical management following a stroke.

70. The maximum score that can be achieved in the ABCD scoring system used to predict the 7-day risk of stroke after a transient ischaemic attack is:
 a 4.
 b 6.
 c 8.
 d 12.

71. Virchow's triad includes all of the following, except:
 a Venous stasis.
 b Injury to veins.
 c Blood hypercoagulability.
 d Venous thrombosis.

72. An urgent carotid endarterectomy is recommended in:
 a Patients with stroke in evolution.
 b Patients with stuttering hemiplegia.
 c Patients with extensive neurological deficits.
 d Patients with a crescendo transient ischaemic attack.

73. Statins work by inhibiting:
 a Absorption of cholesterol.
 b Transport of cholesterol.
 c Cholesterol biosynthesis.
 d All of the above.

74. The diagnostic investigation of choice for pulmonary embolism is:
    a CT scan.
    b MRI.
    c Contrast MRI.
    d Ventilation perfusion scan.

75. The artery that is most commonly affected by atherosclerosis is the:
    a Superficial femoral artery.
    b Popliteal artery.
    c Anterior tibial artery.
    d Aortic bifurcation.

76. A 65-year-old patient with a past history of smoking and hypertension and a history of intermittent pain in the right leg for 6 months is referred by a general practitioner. The pain is worse after walking a short distance and on standing for prolonged periods. The pain is relieved by sitting down and lying down. The most likely cause of the pain is:
    a Intermittent claudication due to peripheral arterial disease.
    b Spinal stenosis.
    c Osteoarthritis of the hip.
    d Prolapsed intervertebral disc with nerve root compression.

77. Diabetic patients on metformin requiring contrast enhanced computed tomography (CT) should stop taking metformin 48 hours before the procedure. The rationale behind this is:
    a To prevent lactic acidosis.
    b To prevent renal failure.
    c To avoid anaphylaxis.
    d To prevent ketoacidosis.

78. A 20-year-old male patient with no significant past medical and family history presents with intermittent claudication in his left calf for 6 months. His angiogram demonstrates narrowing at the right external iliac artery. The most likely cause is:
    a Buerger's disease.
    b Cystic adventitial disease.
    c Fibromuscular dysplasia.
    d Atherosclerosis.

79. The procedure of choice in patients with iliac artery stenosis is:
    a Angioplasty.
    b Iliac stenting.
    c Aorto-iliac revascularisation.
    d Medical therapy.

80. The procedure of choice in patients with iliac artery occlusion is:
    a Angioplasty.
    b Iliac stenting.
    c Aorto-iliac revascularisation.
    d Medical therapy.

81. A 58-year-old male patient presenting with intermittent claudication in his left calf is diagnosed with popliteal artery stenosis. His claudication distance is getting worse and at present he can barely walk up to 50 yards. He is already on maximal medical therapy. The most preferred treatment of choice is:
    a Angioplasty.
    b Femoropopliteal bypass.
    c Stenting.
    d None of the above.

82. A 45-year-old businessman with a history of progressive claudication in his right leg is diagnosed with complete superficial femoral artery occlusion on CT angiogram. The preferred treatment of choice for this patient is:
    a Angioplasty.
    b Ileofemoral bypass.
    c Stenting.
    d Medical therapy.

83. The ankle brachial pressure index is the most useful non-invasive investigation in patients with peripheral vascular disease. However, it may be falsely elevated in one of the following conditions:
    a Diabetes.
    b Hypertension.
    c Following femoropopliteal bypass.
    d Varicose veins.

84. The antihypertensive drug of choice in patients with peripheral arterial disease is:
   a ACE inhibitors.
   b β-blockers.
   c Calcium-channel blockers.
   d Bendroflumethiazide.

85. Cilostazol is a phosphodiesterase III inhibitor and it has been shown to significantly improve maximal and pain-free walking distance in patients with intermittent claudication. It has all of the following properties, except:
   a Vasodilatation.
   b Anti-thrombotic.
   c Anti-platelet.
   d Anti-cholesterol.

86. Diabetic foot ulcers are:
   a Neuropathic in origin.
   b Ischaemic in origin.
   c Neuro-ischaemic in origin.
   d Infective in origin.

87. The most common organism causing infection in patients with diabetic foot ulcer is:
   a *Escherichia coli.*
   b *Pseudomonas* species.
   c *Staphylococcus aureus.*
   d *Clostridium* species.

88. The most common cause of acute lower limb ischaemia is:
   a Embolism associated with atrial fibrillation.
   b Thrombosis secondary to atherosclerosis.
   c Mural thrombosis associated with acute myocardial infarction.
   d Anti-phospholipid syndrome.

89. All of the following are contraindications for thrombolytic therapy, except:
   a Stroke within the last 2 months.
   b Active internal bleeding.
   c Pregnancy.
   d Vascular surgery within the last 6 weeks.

90. The preferred thrombolytic drug of choice in patients with acute critical limb ischaemia is:
    a Tissue plasminogen activator (tPA).
    b Streptokinase.
    c Urokinase.
    d Heparin.

91. A 40-year-old male patient presents with a 6-hour history of sudden onset of pain in the right leg. There is no significant past medical history. On clinical examination he has an irregularly irregular pulse with a pulse rate of 130/min, and pulseless, pale right leg with loss of sensation. He is taken to theatre for exploration of the right femoral artery. A 5 cm embolus is removed and a check angiogram shows occlusion of the popliteal artery. The most appropriate next step in the management of this patient is:
    a Operative angioplasty.
    b Popliteal embolectomy.
    c Operative thrombolysis.
    d Distal bypass.

92. The risk of mortality in patients with acute ischaemic limb due to embolism is high. All of the following are underlying risk factors, except:
    a Poor cardiac function.
    b Associated peripheral vascular disease.
    c Long duration of symptoms.
    d Need for amputation.

93. A 25-year-old male patient involved in a road traffic incident is brought into A&E. On arrival, he is complaining of central chest pain. On examination, he is conscious with a GCS of 15/15 and other observations were normal. He is tender over the manubrium sterni. As a part of trauma series a chest X-ray is taken which shows depression of the left main stem bronchus and associated widening of the mediastinum >8 cm. The next appropriate step in the management of this patient is:
    a Angiography.
    b Spiral computed tomography of the chest.
    c Thoracotomy.
    d Repeat chest X-ray 24 hours later.

94. Which one of the following features is not a hard sign of vascular injury requiring exploration?
a History of severe bleeding.
b Absent distal pulses.
c Expanding haematoma.
d Signs of acute ischaemia.

95. A 35-year-old male patient presents with active bleeding from the right groin after being involved in a road traffic incident. Following fluid resuscitation he is taken to theatre for exploration of the right groin. At exploration more than 50% of the circumference of the superficial femoral artery is damaged. The best way to repair the artery is:
a Excision of the damaged area and end-to-end anastomosis.
b Direct suture repair.
c Ligation above the damaged area and an ileofemoral bypass.
d Repair using a prosthetic graft.

96. The preferred diagnostic modality for the evaluation of zone II vascular injuries of the neck is:
a Duplex Doppler.
b Ultrasound examination.
c Angiography.
d CT scan.

97. A 60-year-old male patient presents with a gunshot wound injury to the right side of the neck. Helical CT angiography shows a thrombosed right-sided vertebral artery with no other vascular injury. The treatment of choice for this patient is:
a Angiography and thrombolysis.
b Thrombectomy and repair.
c No further treatment is required, if patient is haemodynamically stable.
d Ligation of the vertebral artery.

98. Which of the following statements regarding subclavian steal syndrome is true?
a There is reversal of blood flow in the ipsilateral vertebral artery.
b There is reversal of blood flow in the contralateral carotid artery.
c There is reversal of blood flow in the contralateral vertebral artery.
d There is bilateral reversal of blood flow in the vertebral arteries.

99. A 50-year-old male, a heavy alcoholic and smoker, presents with a 3-hour history of increasing shortness of breath. He started having this pain while eating, which is constant and radiates to the back and interscapular region. He is a known hypertensive. On examination, he is cold and clammy with a heart rate of 130/min and BP of 80/40 mmHg. JVP is normal. All peripheral pulses are present and equal. Breath sounds are decreased at the left lung base and chest X-ray shows left pleural effusion. Which one of the following is the most likely diagnosis?
    a Acute aortic dissection.
    b Acute myocardial infarction.
    c Rupture of the oesophagus.
    d Acute pulmonary embolism.

100. The most likely diagnosis in a patient with local gigantism of the leg associated with increased pulsation of the lower limb veins is:
    a Soft tissue sarcoma.
    b Arteriovenous fistula.
    c Varicose veins.
    d Incompetence of the saphenofemoral junction.

101. Which one of the following is not a feature of arterial occlusion?
    a Cyanosis.
    b Pallor.
    c Paralysis.
    d Paraesthesia.

102. Sympathectomy is effective in all of the following conditions, except:
    a Intermittent claudication.
    b Hyperhidrosis.
    c Raynaud's disease.
    d Causalgia.

103. Mycotic aneurysms are secondary to:
    a Fungal infection.
    b Blood borne infection (intravascular).
    c Infection introduced from outside (extravascular).
    d Both intravascular and extravascular infection.

104. Neo-intimal hyperplasia causes vascular graft failure as a result of hypertrophy of:
a Endothelial cells.
b Collagen fibres.
c Smooth muscle cells.
d Elastic fibres.

105. All of the following statements about axillary vein thrombosis are correct, except:
a It may be caused by a cervical rib.
b It is treated with intravenous anticoagulant.
c Embolectomy is performed in all cases.
d It may occur following excessive exercise.

106. All of the following statements regarding AV fistula are correct, except:
a It causes arterialisation of the veins.
b Proximal compression causes an increase in heart rate.
c It causes LV enlargement and LVF.
d None of the above.

107. Which of the following statements regarding intermittent claudication is incorrect?
a It appears as a cramp-like pain.
b It can occur when sitting for a long time in a cramped position.
c If it occurs in an upper limb, it is known as writer's spasm.
d It is relieved by rest.

108. Bilateral pulseless disease in the upper limbs is caused by:
a Aorto-arteritis.
b Co-arctation of the aorta.
c Fibromuscular dysplasia.
d Buerger's disease.

109. The best indication for lumbar sympathectomy in Buerger's disease is:
a Pain at rest.
b Intermittent claudication.
c Ulceration of the foot.
d Gangrene of the foot.

110. Aorto-iliac occlusion is characterised by:
a Backache.
b Hypoanaesthesia.
c Gangrene of the toes.
d Impotence.
e All of the above.

111. The earliest clinical feature associated with upper limb ischaemia is:
a Pain on passive hyperextension of the fingers.
b Claudication.
c Gangrene of the fingers.
d Pain at rest.

112. The sympathetic ganglia spared in lumbar sympathectomy is:
a L_1.
b L_2.
c L_3.
d L_4.

Answers: Vascular surgery

1. **d** All of the above.

2. **c** Port wine stains.

3. **a** AV malformations are direct arteriovenous communications.

4. **d** Gastric ulcer.

5. **d** All of the above.

6. **d** Ethiodol.

7. **b** Ruptured popliteal cyst.

8. **d** Lymphoedema praecox.

9. **a** 6 months.

10. **c** 6 months.

11. **b** Venous duplex scan.

12. **a** Medial aspect of lower leg.

13. **b** Pain relief immediately after the cessation of exercise.

14. **b** 25–35 mmHg.

15. **d** Class IV.

16. a Lower limb venous disease.

17. a Chronic venous insufficiency.

18. d Saphenous nerve.

19. b Common peroneal nerve.

20. a Sural nerve.

21. c It does not treat the varices.

22. a Pressure application and elevation of the leg.

23. c Internal jugular vein.

24. a It provides a direct route to the superior vena cava.

25. d Can be used as soon as the wounds have healed.

26. a Deep vein thrombosis.

27. a Stenosis.

28. a Angioplasty.

29. d 4–6 weeks.

30. c 10%.

31. a Radiocephalic fistula.

32. b Thrombosis of the superior mesenteric artery.

33. a Radial artery.

34. b Chronic mesenteric ischaemia.

35. c Atherosclerosis.

36. d Splenic artery.

37. c Endovascular repair.

38. c Endoleak.

39. b Turner syndrome.

40. b Endovascular repair.

41. a Isthmus of the aorta.

42. a It is six times more common in women.

43. a 75% of patients are symptomatic at the time of diagnosis.

44. b Ultrasound.

45. d 1.1%.

46. a <2%.

47. b 6 months.

48. d Patients with low/absent urine output.

49. b Size of aneurysm.

50. d >4cm.

51. b Popliteal.

52. b >75% are bilateral.

53. d An inlay graft repair.

54. d An inlay graft repair.

55. a Nifedipine.

56. b β-blockers.

57. a Pallor, cyanosis, rubor.

58. a It commonly affects men.

59. d Acute hypercellular occlusive thrombus.

60. a Small and medium arteries of the distal limb.

61. c Smoking.

62. a Temporal arteritis.

63. a Corticosteroids.

64. d All of the above.

65. d C8, T1 nerve roots.

66. c Neurological symptoms.

67. a Thromboembolism of the internal carotid artery.

68. d Homonymous hemianopia.

69. a 7-day risk of stroke after a transient ischaemic attack.

70. b 6.

71. b Injury to veins.

72. a Patients with stroke in evolution.

73. d All of the above.

74. d Ventilation perfusion scan.

75. a Superficial femoral artery.

76. b Spinal stenosis.

77. a To prevent lactic acidosis.

78. c Fibromuscular dysplasia.

79. a Angioplasty.

80. b Iliac stenting.

81. a Angioplasty.

82. b Ileofemoral bypass.

83. a Diabetes.

84. a ACE inhibitors.

85. d Anti-cholesterol.

86. a Neuropathic in origin.

87. c *Staphylococcus aureus.*

88. b Thrombosis secondary to atherosclerosis.

89. d Vascular surgery within the last 6 weeks.

90. a Tissue plasminogen activator (tPA).

91. c Operative thrombolysis.

92. c Long duration of symptoms.

93. b Spiral computed tomography of the chest.

94. a History of severe bleeding.

95. a Excision of the damaged area and end-to-end anastomosis.

96. a Duplex Doppler.

97. c No further treatment is required, if patient is haemodynamically stable.

98. a There is reversal of blood flow in the ipsilateral vertebral artery.

99. c Rupture of the oesophagus.

100. b Arteriovenous fistula.

101. a Cyanosis.

102. a Intermittent claudication.

103. b Blood borne infection (intravascular).

104. c Smooth muscle cells.

105. c Embolectomy is performed in all cases.

106. b Proximal compression causes an increase in heart rate.

107. b It can occur when sitting for a long time in a cramped position.

108. a Aorto-arteritis.

109. a Pain at rest.

110. e All of the above.

111. a Pain on passive hyperextension of the fingers.

112. a L_1.

7
Breast surgery

Questions

1. Which one of the following statements with regard to breast cancer is incorrect?
   a 5% of breast cancers are sporadic.
   b Life-time risk is one in nine.
   c It is uncommon below the age of 35 years.
   d BRCA-1 and BRCA-2 genetic defects are the most common genetic abnormality.

2. A 34-year-old female presents with a 2-month history of a painful right breast lump. Pain is mainly during menstruation. There is no significant past medical history or family history of breast cancer. Clinical examination reveals a diffuse lump in her right breast. The investigation of choice for the further evaluation of the lump is:
   a Ultrasound.
   b Mammogram.
   c Magnetic resonance imaging (MRI).
   d Ultrasound Doppler.

3. Which of the following statements regarding mammographic examination is incorrect?
   a The sensitivity of mammogram for detection of breast cancer is age dependent.
   b The denser the breast the more effective the mammogram.
   c Mammography is rarely indicated in women under the age of 35 years.
   d None of the above.

4. The investigation of choice for early detection of breast cancer in patients with breast implants is:
   a Magnetic resonance imaging (MRI).
   b CT scan.
   c Ultrasound.
   d Mammogram.

5. The investigation of choice in a patient with suspected recurrence following breast conservation surgery is:
   a Magnetic resonance imaging (MRI).
   b CT scan.
   c Ultrasound.
   d Mammogram.

6. Which of the following findings on magnetic resonance imaging (MRI) does not require further evaluation?
   a Well-defined mass.
   b Clustered micro-calcification.
   c Architectural distortion.
   d Spiculated lesion.

7. The best screening test for females aged between 32–39 years with a high risk of breast cancer is:
   a Magnetic resonance imaging (MRI).
   b CT scan.
   c Ultrasound.
   d Mammogram.

8. The sampling technique of choice in a patient with a suspicious breast lesion on mammography and ultrasound is:
   a FNAC.
   b Core biopsy.
   c Stereotactic core biopsy.
   d Vacuum-assisted mammotomy.

9. The sampling technique of choice in a patient with a suspicious breast lesion detected by mammography but not visible on ultrasound is:
   a FNAC.
   b Core biopsy.
   c Stereotactic core biopsy.
   d Vacuum-assisted mammotomy.

10. The parameter that is not used in the calculation of the Nottingham prognostic index is:
    a Tumour grade.
    b Lymphovascular invasion.
    c Tumour size.
    d Lymph node status.

11. A 52-year-old female underwent breast conservation surgery and axillary nodal clearance. The histology shows a 3 cm, well-differentiated, intraductal carcinoma. Three out of 15 lymph nodes are involved by the tumour. The Nottingham prognostic index for this patient is:
    a 4.4.
    b 3.6.
    c 5.2.
    d 6.

12. All of the following except one is not an independent prognostic factor for breast cancer:
    a Lymph node status.
    b Histological grade.
    c Size of the tumour.
    d Estrogen receptor status.

13. Which of the following is not seen in Paget's disease of the breast?
    a Eczematous skin lesions.
    b Intraductal invasive carcinoma.
    c Early lymph node metastasis.
    d Multifocal invasive carcinoma.

14. A contraindication for breast conservation surgery is:
    a 3 cm lesion in the left upper outer quadrant.
    b Multifocal disease.
    c 2 cm lesion located centrally in a large breast.
    d 3 cm lesion in the right upper quadrant with a family history of breast cancer.

15. The preferred breast conservation surgical option is:
    a Quadrantectomy.
    b Wide local excision.
    c Local excision.
    d Lumpectomy.

16. All of the following factors except one affect the incidence of local recurrence following breast conservation surgery:
    a Tumour grade.
    b Lymphovascular invasion.
    c Size of the tumour.
    d Hormone receptor status.

17. Which one of the following statements with regard to local recurrence following breast conservation surgery is incorrect?
    a Recurrence within 5 years is associated with worst outcome.
    b Presence of an extensive in situ component is associated with an increased risk of local recurrence.
    c Local recurrence is more common in elderly patients.
    d Radiotherapy reduces the incidence of local recurrence.

18. The breast is embryologically derived from:
    a Sweat gland.
    b Sebaceous gland.
    c Subcutaneous fat.
    d Pectoral fascia.

✓ 19. Which one of the following statements with regard to lymph node staging of breast cancer is incorrect?
    a Sentinel lymph node biopsy is the procedure of choice in the absence of palpable lymph nodes.
    b The majority of patients with ductal carcinoma in situ should not have axillary surgery.
    c Physical examination is associated with a high false positive and false negative rate.
    d Axillary lymph node dissection improves overall survival significantly.

20. The motor nerves that are at risk of injury during axillary lymph node dissection are the:
    a Medial pectoral nerve, long thoracic nerve of Bell, thoracodorsal nerve.
    b Intercostobrachial nerve, lateral pectoral nerve, long thoracic nerve of Bell.
    c Intercostobrachial nerve, medial pectoral nerve, thoracodorsal nerve.
    d Lateral pectoral nerve, long thoracic nerve of Bell, thoracodorsal nerve.

21. Damage to which of the following nerves results in winging of the scapula?
    a Thoracodorsal nerve.
    b Long thoracic nerve of Bell.
    c Medial pectoral nerve.
    d Lateral pectoral nerve.

22. A 50-year-old female with a 2 cm palpable breast lesion and clinically negative axillary lymph node is confirmed to have an invasive breast carcinoma on ultrasound core biopsy. The appropriate lymph node staging method in this patient is:
    a Sentinel lymph node biopsy at the time of breast conservation surgery.
    b Axillary lymph node sampling.
    c Axillary lymph node dissection.
    d Ultrasound guided axillary lymph node biopsy.

23. Sentinel lymph node biopsy is not recommended in patients with:
    a Invasive cancer of less than 5 cm.
    b Ductal carcinoma in situ presenting with a palpable mass.
    c Previous axillary surgery.
    d 4 cm lesion in the centre of the breast.

24. Sentinel lymph node biopsy is not recommended in patients with the following conditions with the exception of:
    a Inflammatory breast cancer.
    b Pregnant females.
    c Multicentric disease.
    d Patients on neoadjuvant therapy.

25. A 45-year-old female with a 3 cm palpable right breast lesion is referred to a breast clinic for further evaluation. On examination, there is a 3 cm hard mass in the right upper quadrant. She is also found to have palpable right axillary lymph nodes. The most appropriate next step in the management is:
    a Ultrasound guided core biopsy of the breast lesion and FNAC of the axillary lymph node.
    b Mammogram and ultrasound of the breast lesion and sentinel lymph node biopsy.
    c US and mammogram followed by core biopsy of the breast lesion and FNAC of the axillary nodes.
    d Wide local excision and sentinel lymph node biopsy.

26. Which of the following factors are independent predictors of invasive cancer in patients with ductal carcinoma in situ (DCIS)?
    a Age <55 years.
    b Mammographic size >4 cm.
    c High-grade disease.
    d Diagnosis made with core biopsy.
    e All of the above.

27. Which one of the following statements regarding BRCA-1 associated breast cancer is false?
    a They are more frequently grade III tumours.
    b They are often estrogen receptor (ER) positive.
    c Medullary carcinomas are more frequent.
    d All of the above.

28. Which one of the following statements with regard to risk reduction mastectomy (RRM) in patients with a family history of BRCA-1 and BRCA-2 mutations is incorrect?
    a RRM reduces the incidence of breast cancer by over 95%.
    b Nipple areolar complex preserving surgery is associated with a higher complication rate.
    c Early reconstruction is not contraindicated if early postoperative radiotherapy is anticipated.
    d It is contraindicated in patients choosing surgery for cosmetic reasons.

29. Immediate breast reconstruction following mastectomy is associated with all of the following advantages, except:
    a Maximal preservation of breast skin.
    b Improved preservation of inframammary fold.
    c Better cosmetic results.
    d Better overall survival.

30. Which one of the following is not a contraindication for breast reconstruction surgery?
    a Unresectable chest wall disease.
    b Multiple serious co-morbidities.
    c Progressive systemic disease.
    d Familial breast cancer.

31. The latissimus dorsi myocutaneous flap is based on blood supply from the:
    a Thoracodorsal artery.
    b Internal mammary artery.
    c Thoracoacromial artery.
    d Suprascapular artery.

32. The common site for the placement of a tissue expander following mastectomy is:
    a Under the chest wall muscle.
    b Under the skin.
    c Posterior to the pectoral fascia.
    d Within the pectoralis major muscle.

33. The common complication following breast implant reconstruction is:
    a Haematoma formation.
    b Seroma formation.
    c Capsular contracture.
    d Flap necrosis.

34. A rectus abdominis muscle flap may rely on its blood supply from all of the following vessels, except the:
    a Deep inferior epigastric artery.
    b Deep superficial epigastric artery.
    c Superficial inferior epigastric artery.
    d Musculophrenic artery.

35. A 25-year-old female presents with a painless lump in her right breast. On examination there is a 2 cm mobile, firm, well-defined mass present in the lower outer quadrant. The most likely diagnosis is:

   a Fibroadenoma.
   b Breast cancer.
   c Phyllodes tumour.
   d Hamartoma.

36. Excision of a fibroadenoma is recommended in which of the following situations:

   a Lesions >4 cm.
   b Rapid increase in size.
   c Lesions causing significant distortion of breast profile.
   d All of the above.

37. The treatment of choice in a patient with a 3.5 cm histologically confirmed fibroadenoma of the breast is:

   a Reassurance.
   b Lumpectomy.
   c Wide local excision.
   d Further follow-up with ultrasound.

38. Phyllodes tumours are characterised by all of the following, except:

   a Age of onset is 15–20 years earlier than fibroadenomas.
   b Less common than fibroadenomas.
   c The majority are benign.
   d Lymph node metastasis is rare.

39. The characteristic features of phyllodes tumour are:

   a Leaf-like appearance on the cut surface.
   b Presence of cutaneous engorgement.
   c High incidence of local recurrence.
   d All of the above.
   e None of the above.

40. The common cause of bloody nipple discharge is:

   a Intraductal papilloma.
   b Nipple adenoma.
   c Ductal carcinoma in situ.
   d Duct ectasia.

41. A 60-year-old female with a 3-month history of bloody nipple discharge and normal clinical and mammographic findings should be managed by:
a   Cytology of nipple discharge.
b   Microdochectomy.
c   Total duct excision.
d   Simple mastectomy.

42. The treatment of choice for a 30-year-old pregnant lady with bloody nipple discharge and normal clinical examination is:
a   Ultrasound breast + biopsy.
b   Reassurance.
c   Microdochectomy.
d   Total duct excision.

43. A 40-year-old female with bilateral cyclical breast pain with no palpable mass on clinical examination is referred to you by her general practitioner. The next step in the management of this patient is:
a   Mammography.
b   Analgesics and reassurance.
c   Tamoxifen.
d   Evening primrose oil.

44. The most effective drug for the treatment of cyclical mastalgia is:
a   Tamoxifen.
b   Danazol.
c   Bromocriptine.
d   Evening primrose oil.

45. A risk factor for peri-ductal mastitis is:
a   Pregnancy.
b   Smoking.
c   Diabetes.
d   Lactation.

46. The organism most commonly responsible for infections during lactation is:
a   *Staphylococcus aureus.*
b   *Streptococcus.*
c   Anaerobes.
d   *Streptococcus milleri.*

47. A 35-year-old female presents with a painful right breast lump during lactation. Clinical examination reveals a tender, non-fluctuating inflammatory mass in the right inner and lower quadrant. The treatment of choice is:

a Incision and drainage.

b Antibiotics followed by ultrasound guided aspiration.

c Antibiotics followed by mammography.

d Antibiotics alone.

48. A 30-year-old female presents with a 3-day history of a painful right breast. There is no significant past medical history. Clinical examination reveals thickened palpable cord-associated erythema over the lower part of the breast. The most likely diagnosis is:

a Mondor's disease.

b Traumatic fat necrosis.

c Locally advanced breast cancer.

d Fibroadenosis.

49. The drug used in the medical management of gynaecomastia is:

a Bromocryptine.

b Danazole.

c Metoclopramide.

d Minocycline.

50. Which one of the following drugs does not cause gynaecomastia?

a Ranitidine.

b Enalapril.

c Diazepam.

d Phenytoin.

e Ciprofloxacin.

51. All of the following are risk factors for local recurrence following breast conservation surgery, except:

a Positive resection margin.

b Grade of tumour.

c Presence of extensive intraductal component.

d None of the above.

52. The most common site of recurrence of invasive breast cancer following mastectomy is:
   a Chest wall.
   b Axilla.
   c Lung.
   d Bone.

53. The patients at high risk of developing loco-regional recurrence are those with:
   a Grade III cancer.
   b Involvement of more than four lymph nodes.
   c Involvement of the pectoral fascia.
   d All of the above.

54. The preferred hormonal therapy in a 65-year-old female with metastatic breast cancer is:
   a Tamoxifen.
   b Letrozole.
   c Progestogen.
   d Chemotherapy.

55. The preferred hormonal treatment in pre-menopausal women with metastatic breast cancer is:
   a Tamoxifen.
   b Aromatase inhibitor.
   c Progestogen.
   d LHRH agonist.

56. The preferred treatment of choice in a patient with estrogen receptor negative metastatic breast cancer is:
   a Trastuzumab.
   b Aromatase inhibitor.
   c Tamoxifen.
   d Chemotherapy.

57. The side-effects of tamoxifen include:
   a Endometrial cancer.
   b Thromboembolism.
   c Hot flushes and vaginal dryness.
   d Weight gain.
   e All of the above.

58. All of the following are risk factors for male breast cancer, except:
    a Obesity.
    b Klinefelter's syndrome.
    c Cirrhosis.
    d Gynaecomastia.

59. Which of the following statements with regard to the epidemiology of male breast cancer is incorrect?
    a It accounts for >10% of all breast cancers in Western countries.
    b The prevalence increases with age.
    c The average age of diagnosis is 10 years younger than in women.
    d 15–20% of patients have a family history of breast cancer.

60. A 55-year-old female presents with an itchy skin lesion around the nipple for the last 6 weeks. On clinical examination she has an eczematous lesion over the areola. Biopsy shows large rounded intra-epidermal cells with abundant clear pale cytoplasm and enlarged pleomorphic and hyperchromatic nuclei. The most likely diagnosis is:
    a Paget's disease.
    b Basal cell carcinoma.
    c Chronic eczema.
    d Malignant melanoma.

61. Which one of the following statements with regard to Paget's disease is incorrect?
    a Over 95% of women have underlying malignancy.
    b Burning, itching and change in the sensation of the nipple and areola is the first symptom.
    c The common reason for delay in diagnosis is due to misdiagnosis as eczema.
    d Prognosis depends on the size of the eczematous lesion.

62. The most common type of male breast cancer is:
    a Invasive lobular carcinoma.
    b Infiltrating ductal carcinoma.
    c Paget's disease.
    d Inflammatory carcinoma.

63. Which one of the following statements with regard to male breast cancer (MBC) is incorrect?
    a The majority of MBCs are invasive carcinomas.
    b MBC has a lower rate of estrogen receptor positivity than female breast cancers.
    c Lobular carcinoma in situ is rare.
    d MBCs have a higher rate of progestogen receptor positivity than female breast cancer.

64. Which of the following statements with regard to ductal carcinoma in situ (DCIS) is incorrect?
    a It accounts for 20–30% of all screen detected tumours.
    b It is a pre-invasive breast cancer.
    c Most of them are multicentric.
    d Screen detected DCISs are frequently small, localised tumours.

65. Lobular carcinoma in situ is:
    a A pre-malignant lesion.
    b A marker of underlying invasive cancer.
    c Often seen in the elderly population.
    d Accounts for ~10% of screen detected tumours.

66. The incidence of macroscopic lymph node involvement in patients with ductal carcinoma in situ (DCIS) is:
    a <10%.
    b <1%.
    c <5%.
    d 5–10%.

67. All of the following are risk factors for the recurrence of ductal carcinoma in situ (DCIS), except:
    a Poorly-differentiated DCIS.
    b High-grade DCIS.
    c Absence of comedo necrosis.
    d Excision margins of less than 1 cm on breast conservation surgery.

68. Tamoxifen is indicated in which one of the following group of patients with ductal carcinoma in situ (DCIS):
   a Estrogen receptor (ER) negative tumours following breast conservation surgery.
   b ER positive tumours following mastectomy.
   c ER and HER-2 positive tumours following mastectomy.
   d ER positive tumours following breast conservation surgery.

69. The long-term use of tamoxifen increases the incidence of which one of the following cancers?
   a Uterine carcinoma.
   b Ovarian cancer.
   c Breast cancer.
   d Cervical cancer.

70. The side-effects of aromatase inhibitors include:
   a Dyspareunia.
   b Bone fracture.
   c Hypercholesterolemia.
   d Joint disorder.
   e All of the above.

71. Which one of the following groups of patients with breast cancer receives the maximum benefit from adjuvant chemotherapy?
   a Breast cancer with lymph node level I, II, III involvement with estrogen receptor (ER) and progestogen receptor (PR) negative.
   b Breast cancer with lymph node I, II, III involvement with HER-2 negative.
   c Age >35 years with ER and PR positive and node negative tumours.
   d Tumour >2 cm, HER-2 positive and node negative.

72. The endocrine treatment of choice in pre-menopausal women with hormone responsive tumours is:
   a Letrozole.
   b Anastrozole.
   c Tamoxifen.
   d Goserelin.

73. A 65-year-old female patient presents with a 6 cm lesion in her right breast associated with local signs of inflammation. It is confirmed as an estrogen receptor (ER) positive, locally advanced breast cancer. This patient should be treated with:
   a Letrozole.
   b Tamoxifen.
   c Systemic therapy.
   d Fulvestrant.

74. In patients with breast cancer, chest wall involvement means involvement of any one of the following structures, except:
   a Serratus anterior.
   b Pectoralis major.
   c Intercostal muscles.
   d Ribs.

75. Increased susceptibility to breast cancer is likely to be associated with a mutation in which of the following genes?
   a p^{53}.
   b BRCA-1.
   c Retinoblastoma (Rb).
   d K-ras.

76. All of the following are features of a malignant breast tumour on a mammogram, except:
   a Spiculation.
   b Microcalcification.
   c Macrocalcification.
   d An irregular mass.

77. Which one of the following is not used in the reconstruction of breast tissue?
   a Transverse rectus abdominis myocutaneous flap.
   b Latissimus dorsi myocutaneous flap.
   c Pectoralis major myocutaneous flap.
   d Transverse rectus abdominis free flap.

78. Green nipple discharge is most commonly seen in which of the following conditions?
    a Duct papilloma.
    b Duct ectasia.
    c Retention cyst.
    d Fibroadenosis.

79. All of the following are risk factors for breast carcinomas, except:
    a Ovarian malignancy.
    b Family history of breast carcinoma.
    c Fibroadenosis.
    d Multiparity.

80. Peau d'orange is due to:
    a Arterial obstruction.
    b Blockage of the subdermal lymphatics.
    c Invasion of the skin with malignant cells.
    d Secondary infection.

81. Cystosarcoma phyllodes is treated by:
    a Simple mastectomy.
    b Radical mastectomy.
    c Modified radical mastectomy.
    d Conservation treatment with antibiotics.

82. The type of mammary ductal carcinoma in situ (DCIS) most likely to result in a palpable abnormality in the breast is:
    a Apocrine DCIS.
    b Neuroendocrine DCIS.
    c Well-differentiated DCIS.
    d Comedo DCIS.

83. In which of the following types of breast carcinoma would you consider biopsy of the opposite breast?
    a Poorly-differentiated adenocarcinoma.
    b Medullary carcinoma.
    c Lobular carcinoma.
    d Comedo carcinoma.

84. The treatment of choice in ductal papilloma of the breast is:
   a Simple mastectomy.
   b Microdochectomy.
   c Local wide excision.
   d Chemotherapy.

85. Mondor's disease is:
   a Thrombophlebitis of the superficial veins of the breast.
   b Carcinoma of the breast.
   c A pre-malignant condition of the breast.
   d Filariasis of the breast.

86. Which histological variant of breast carcinoma is multicentric and bilateral?
   a Ductal carcinoma.
   b Lobular carcinoma.
   c Mucoid carcinoma.
   d Colloid carcinoma.

87. Which of the following breast cancers carries the best prognosis?
   a Ductal carcinoma.
   b Lobular carcinoma.
   c Adenoid cystic carcinoma.
   d Colloid carcinoma.

88. Which of the following statements regarding Cooper's ligaments is true?
   a They are fibrous bands between the breast skin and subcutaneous tissue.
   b They are fibrous bands between the breast skin and pectoralis fascia.
   c They are thickened sub-dermal breast lymphatics.
   d They are fibrous bands between the skin and the clavipectoral fascia.

89. Peau d'orange in breast cancer is indicative of:
   a Tumour growth under the skin.
   b Infiltration of Cooper's ligaments.
   c Involvement of the dermal and subdermal lymphatics.
   d Low grade secondary infection.

90. The most common site of bony metastasis in breast carcinoma is the:
    a Cervical vertebra.
    b Thoracic vertebra.
    c Lumbar vertebra.
    d Sacral vertebra.

91. Pectoralis minor is supplied by the:
    a Lateral pectoral nerve.
    b Medial pectoral nerve.
    c Medial and lateral pectoral nerves.
    d Nerve to pectoralis minor.

92. Latissimus dorsi is supplied by the:
    a Thoracodorsal nerve.
    b Long thoracic nerve of Bell.
    c Suprascapular nerve.
    d Radial nerve.

93. A quadrangular space lies between the subscapularis muscle and the teres major muscle in the posterior wall of the axilla. It is bounded laterally by the humerus and medially by the long head of the triceps. Which of the following structures is not transmitted through this space?
    a The radial nerve.
    b The axillary nerve.
    c The posterior circumflex artery.
    d The posterior circumflex vein.

94. The skin of axilla is supplied by the:
    a Musculocutaneous nerve.
    b Intercostobrachial nerve.
    c Nerve to pectoralis major.
    d Nerve to serratus anterior.

Answers: Breast surgery

1. a 5% of breast cancers are sporadic.

2. a Ultrasound.

3. b The denser the breast the more effective the mammogram.

4. a Magnetic resonance imaging (MRI).

5. a Magnetic resonance imaging (MRI).

6. a Well-defined mass.

7. a Magnetic resonance imaging (MRI).

8. b Core biopsy.

9. c Stereotactic core biopsy.

10. b Lymphovascular invasion.

11. a 4.4.

12. d Estrogen receptor status.

13. c Early lymph node metastasis.

14. b Multifocal disease.

15. b Wide local excision.

16. d Hormone receptor status.

17. c Local recurrence is more common in elderly patients.

18. a Sweat gland.

19. d Axillary lymph node dissection improves overall survival significantly.

20. a Medial pectoral nerve, long thoracic nerve of Bell, thoracodorsal nerve.

21. b Long thoracic nerve of Bell.

22. a Sentinel lymph node biopsy at the time of breast conservation surgery.

23. c Previous axillary surgery.

24. c Multicentric disease.

25. c US and mammogram followed by core biopsy of the breast lesion and FNAC of the axillary nodes.

26. e All of the above.

27. b They are often estrogen receptor (ER) positive.

28. c Early reconstruction is not contraindicated if early post-operative radiotherapy is anticipated.

29. d Better overall survival.

30. d Familial breast cancer.

31. a Thoracodorsal artery.

32. a Under the chest wall muscle.

33. c Capsular contracture.

34. d Musculophrenic artery.

35. a Fibroadenoma.

36. d All of the above.

37. a Reassurance.

38. a Age of onset is 15–20 years earlier than fibroadenomas.

39. d All of the above.

40. a Intraductal papilloma.

41. c Total duct excision.

42. b Reassurance.

43. a Mammography.

44. a Tamoxifen.

45. b Smoking.

46. a *Staphylococcus aureus.*

47. b Antibiotics followed by ultrasound guided aspiration.

48. a Mondor's disease.

49. b Danazole.

50. e Ciprofloxacin.

51. d None of the above.

52. a Chest wall.

53. d All of the above.

54. b Letrozole.

55. a Tamoxifen.

56. d Chemotherapy.

57. e All of the above.

58. d Gynaecomastia.

59. a It accounts for >10% of all breast cancers in Western countries.

60. a Paget's disease.

61. d Prognosis depends on the size of the eczematous lesion.

62. b Infiltrating ductal carcinoma.

63. b MBC has a lower rate of estrogen receptor positivity than female breast cancers.

64. c Most of them are multicentric.

65. b A marker of underlying invasive cancer.

66. b <1%.

67. c Absence of comedo necrosis.

68. d ER positive tumours following breast conservation surgery.

69. a Uterine carcinoma.

70. e All of the above.

71. a Breast cancer with lymph node level I, II, III involvement with estrogen receptor (ER) and progestogen receptor (PR) negative.

72. c Tamoxifen.

73. a Letrozole.

74. b Pectoralis major.

75. b BRCA-1.

76. c Macrocalcification.

77. c Pectoralis major myocutaneous flap.

78. b Duct ectasia.

79. d Multiparity.

80. b Blockage of the subdermal lymphatics.

81. a Simple mastectomy.

82. d Comedo DCIS.

83. c Lobular carcinoma.

84. b Microdochectomy.

85. a Thrombophlebitis of the superficial veins of the breast.

86. b Lobular carcinoma.

87. d Colloid carcinoma.

88. b They are fibrous bands between the breast skin and pectoralis fascia.

89. c Involvement of the dermal and subdermal lymphatics.

90. c Lumbar vertebra.

91. c Medial and lateral pectoral nerves.

92. a Thoracodorsal nerve.

93. a The radial nerve.

94. b Intercostobrachial nerve.

8
General and emergency surgery

Questions

1. The vasopressor of choice in patients with septic shock is:
   a Noradrenaline.
   b Adrenaline.
   c Dopamine.
   d Dopexamine.

2. The preferred definite airway in a patient with suspected fracture of the larynx and failed endotracheal intubation is:
   a Surgical cricothyroidotomy.
   b Tracheostomy.
   c Needle cricothyroidotomy.
   d None of the above.

3. The oxyhaemoglobin dissociation curve is shifted towards the right by all of the following factors, except:
   a ↑ pH.
   b ↑ temperature.
   c ↑ CO_2.
   d ↑ 2, 3 DPG.

4. Cardiac output is determined by which of the following factors:
   a Preload.
   b Systemic vascular resistance.
   c Myocardial contractility.
   d All of the above.
   e a and b.

5. Preload is determined by all of the following factors, except:
   a Venous capacitance.
   b Peripheral vascular resistance.
   c Volume status.
   d The difference between mean venous and right atrial pressure.

6. A 36-year-old woman was ejected from her car during a head-on collision with a truck. On arrival to A&E her pulse rate is 120/min, blood pressure 80/60 mmHg and she has engorged neck veins. Her chest is clear with equal and good air entry on both sides on auscultation. The most likely diagnosis is:
   a Haemothorax.
   b Tension pneumothorax.
   c Cardiac tamponade.
   d Neurogenic shock.

7. The following feature is useful in the differentiation of neurogenic from cardiogenic shock:
   a Altered consciousness.
   b Decreased urine output.
   c Hypotension without tachycardia.
   d Hypoxia.

8. The most common cause of shock in a trauma patient is:
   a Haemorrhagic shock.
   b Septic shock.
   c Neurogenic shock.
   d Cardiogenic shock.

9. The normal blood volume of a 70 kg adult male is:
   a 7% of body weight.
   b 15% of body weight.
   c 5% of body weight.
   d 10% of body weight.

10. A 23-year-old male is brought into A&E after being stabbed in the left upper quadrant by a rival gang member. On arrival he is anxious and confused, his pulse rate is 140/min, blood pressure 80/60 mmHg, respiration rate 30/min and urine output 5–15 mL/hour. The approximate amount of blood loss in this patient is:
   a 500–750 mL.
   b 750–1,500 mL.
   c 1,500–2,000 mL.
   d >2,000 mL.

11. A 30-year-old male driver of a car involved in a road traffic incident is brought into A&E. On arrival he is anxious with a pulse rate of 120/min, BP 80/50 mmHg and respiratory rate 30/min. He is given 2 litres of crystalloids after which his blood pressure improves to 110/70 mmHg and his pulse rate to 100/min. The A&E team decide to transfuse him. The type of blood that can be used in this scenario is:
   a Fully cross-matched blood.
   b Type specific blood.
   c O- blood.
   d O+ blood.

12. A simple and reliable measure that helps in the identification of adequate tissue perfusion in a shock patient is:
   a Central venous pressure.
   b Urine output.
   c Normalisation of tachycardia.
   d Mean arterial pressure.

13. A pronounced increase in central venous pressure can be caused by all of the following conditions, except:
   a Cardiac tamponade.
   b Tension pneumothorax.
   c Massive blood transfusion.
   d Neurogenic shock.

14. The most common site used for intra-osseus infusion in children is the:
   a Iliac crest.
   b Anterio-medial surface of the proximal tibia.
   c Greater trochanter.
   d Neck of the humerus.

15. Which of the following radiographs are not included as part of trauma series?
    a X-ray of the chest.
    b X-ray of the pelvis.
    c X-ray of the cervical spine.
    d X-ray of the abdomen.

16. In a patient with suspected urethral injury, urethral integrity should be confirmed by which one of the following investigations before insertion of a urinary catheter?
    a Retrograde urethrogram.
    b Computed tomography.
    c Voiding cystourethrogram.
    d Ultrasound of abdomen.

17. A 30-year-old male patient with a flail chest is intubated and considered for transfer to the nearest trauma centre for further management. The proper position of the endotracheal tube should be confirmed by:
    a Arterial blood gas analysis.
    b Capnography.
    c Chest X-ray.
    d Pulse oximetry.

18. Which of the following tests is useful in the confirmation of the location of the endotracheal tube?
    a Arterial blood gas analysis.
    b Pulse oximetry.
    c Capnography.
    d Electrocardiography.

19. Pulse oximetry does not measure:
    a Partial pressure of oxygen.
    b Partial pressure of carbon dioxide.
    c Oxygen saturation of haemoglobin.
    d a and b.

20. A simple, non-invasive test that is useful in the detection of intra-abdominal fluid in trauma patients is:
    a Diagnostic peritoneal lavage.
    b Focused abdominal sonography for trauma (FAST) scan.
    c CT scan.
    d X-ray of abdomen.

21. The best way to provide oxygenation to a patient with facial trauma is:
    a Laryngeal mask.
    b Endotracheal intubation.
    c Oral airway.
    d Nasopharyngeal airway.

22. Which of the following describe the complications associated with positive pressure ventilation?
    a ↑ cardiac output, ↑ preload, ↑ peripheral vascular resistance, ↓ afterload.
    b ↑ cardiac output, ↑ preload, ↓ peripheral vascular resistance, ↓ afterload.
    c ↑ cardiac output, ↓ preload, ↑ peripheral vascular resistance, ↓ afterload.
    d ↓ cardiac output, ↑ preload, ↓ peripheral vascular resistance, ↑ afterload.

23. Which one of the following is not a definitive airway?
    a Tracheostomy.
    b Nasopharyngeal intubation.
    c Laryngeal mask.
    d Endotracheal intubation.

24. A 25-year-old male with head injury following a road traffic accident is brought into A&E. On examination, he has a cervical collar in situ. He is talking inappropriately, opening his eyes and able to move both lower limbs following painful stimuli. The best method to secure the airway in this patient is:
    a Laryngeal mask.
    b Endotracheal intubation.
    c Laryngeal airway.
    d Multilumen oesophageal airway.

25. Which one of the following statements with regard to epigastric hernia is incorrect?
   a The majority are symptomatic.
   b It is more common in males.
   c Incarceration of intra-abdominal viscera is extremely rare.
   d Spontaneous resolution occurs in children under 10 years of age.

26. Which one of the following statements with regard to infantile umbilical hernia is incorrect?
   a 90% disappear by 2 years of age.
   b The majority require surgical repair.
   c Hernias with a defect of >1.5 cm are unlikely to heal spontaneously.
   d Complications are rare.

27. Umbilical hernia in adults is:
   a Common in males.
   b Associated with high morbidity and mortality.
   c Surgical repair is required in almost all patients.
   d b and c.

28. The risk factors for umbilical hernia include all of the following, except:
   a Obesity.
   b Cirrhosis.
   c Peritoneal dialysis.
   d Diabetes.

29. The superficial inguinal ring is situated:
   a Midway between the pubic tubercle and the anterior superior iliac spine.
   b 1 cm above the pubic tubercle.
   c Midway between the pubic symphysis and the anterior superior iliac spine.
   d 1 cm above the pubic symphysis.

30. The deep inguinal ring is a defect in which of the following layers of the abdominal wall?
   a External oblique aponeurosis.
   b Internal oblique aponeurosis.
   c Transversalis fascia.
   d Transversus abdominis muscle.

31. The deep inguinal ring is situated:
    a 1 cm above the midpoint between the pubic tubercle and the anterior superior iliac spine.
    b 1 cm above the midpoint between the pubic symphysis and the anterior superior iliac spine.
    c 1 cm below the midpoint between the pubic symphysis and the anterior superior iliac spine.
    d 1 cm above and lateral to the pubic tubercle.

32. The anterior boundary of the inguinal canal is formed by:
    a External oblique aponeurosis and conjoint tendon.
    b Transversalis fascia and conjoint tendon.
    c Conjoint tendon.
    d Ileopubic tract and inguinal ligament.

33. The relationship between the direct inguinal hernia and the inferior epigastric artery is:
    a Inferior epigastric artery is lateral to the direct hernia.
    b Inferior epigastric artery is medial to the direct hernia.
    c Inferior epigastric artery is anterior to the direct hernia.
    d Inferior epigastric artery is posterior to the direct hernia.

34. Which one of the following statements with regard to inguinal hernia in infants is incorrect?
    a Herniotomy is the treatment of choice.
    b More than half are bilateral.
    c All patients should be offered surgery.
    d Undescended/ectopic testis is associated with inguinal hernia.

35. The most common hernia in females is:
    a Inguinal hernia.
    b Femoral hernia.
    c Epigastric hernia.
    d Lumbar hernia.

36. A 60-year-old male patient with chronic renal failure on peritoneal dialysis presents with an inguinal hernia. The most likely cause of the hernia is:
    a The presence of patent process vaginalis.
    b Weakness of the anterior abdominal wall.
    c Raised intra-abdominal pressure due to peritoneal dialysis.
    d None of the above.

37. The preferred method of repair for a recurrent inguinal hernia is:
   a Lichtenstein repair.
   b Laparoscopic repair.
   c Shouldice repair.
   d McVay repair.

38. A 50-year-old male patient with a right-sided inguinal hernia is booked for a day case hernia repair under local anaesthesia. At the time of consent for the procedure, the patient tells the surgical registrar that he is on warfarin for recurrent deep vein thrombosis. International normalised ratio (INR) is 2.5 on the day of surgery. The best management option for this patient is:
   a Hernia repair as planned.
   b Fresh frozen plasma followed by hernia repair on the same day.
   c Intravenous vitamin K followed by surgical repair on the following day.
   d Surgery should be cancelled and the patient should be admitted later after stopping warfarin for 72 hours.

39. The boundaries of the femoral ring include all of the following, except the:
   a Inguinal ligament.
   b Iliopectineal ligament.
   c Lacunar ligament.
   d Pubic tubercle.

40. The medial boundary of the femoral triangle is formed by the:
   a Pectineus muscle.
   b Adductor magnus.
   c Sartorius.
   d Femoral vein.

41. The most medial structure in the femoral triangle is the:
   a Femoral ring.
   b Femoral vein.
   c Femoral artery.
   d Femoral nerve.

42. The incidence of femoral hernia increases with age. This is most likely due to:
    a Muscle atrophy.
    b Loss of fat.
    c Laxity of the inguinal ligament.
    d High incidence of co-morbidities.

43. The optimal ratio between suture and wound length that is associated with a lower rate of incisional hernia is:
    a 4:1.
    b 5:1.
    c 2:1.
    d 1:1.

44. All of the following are risk factors for the development of an incisional hernia, except:
    a Advanced age.
    b Anaemia.
    c Morbid obesity.
    d Wound infection.

45. In perforation peritonitis free sub-diaphragmatic gas on an erect chest X-ray is seen approximately in:
    a <10%.
    b >70%.
    c 90%.
    d 25%.

46. The factor associated with increased morbidity and mortality following a perforated peptic ulcer is:
    a Young age.
    b Pre-operative hypotension.
    c Duration of pain.
    d C-reactive protein of >100.

47. The surgical treatment of choice in a patient with a perforated duodenal ulcer is:
    a Omental patch closure and peritoneal lavage.
    b Omental patch closure and highly selective vagotomy.
    c Truncal vagotomy and distal gastrectomy.
    d Truncal vagotomy and omental patch repair.

48. Bleeding in disseminated intravascular coagulation is most closely related to:
   a Raised fibrin degradation product level in the blood.
   b Prolonged prothrombin time.
   c Low serum fibrinogen level.
   d Raised thrombin time.

49. The most common cause of upper gastrointestinal bleeding is:
   a Peptic ulcer disease.
   b Oesophageal varices.
   c Oesophagitis.
   d Gastric cancer.

50. Which one of the following parameters is not included in the calculation of the Rockall score?
   a Age.
   b Cause of bleeding.
   c Co-morbidities.
   d Site of bleeding.

51. A 65-year-old female patient with a history of ischaemic heart disease presents with an acute upper gastrointestinal bleed. On examination her pulse rate is 100/min and systolic BP 100 mmHg. Upper GI endoscopy reveals a duodenal ulcer in the first part of the duodenum with an adherent clot. The Rockall score for this patient is:
   a 8.
   b 3.
   c 7.
   d 5.

52. Pre-endoscopic treatment with proton pump inhibitors is recommended in patients with upper gastrointestinal haemorrhage because:
   a It reduces the risk of active bleeding at the time of endoscopy.
   b It reduces the risk of re-bleeding.
   c It reduces the risk of aspiration.
   d It reduces the risk of surgery.

53. The most common site of a bleeding duodenal ulcer is the:
    a Inferior and superior wall of the first part of the duodenum.
    b Posterior wall of the first part of the duodenum.
    c Anterior wall of the first part of the duodenum.
    d Second part of the duodenum.

54. All of the following endoscopic features suggest a high risk of re-bleeding, except:
    a Presence of an adherent clot.
    b Visible vessel.
    c Spurting vessel.
    d Ulcer with a clean base.

55. The majority of patients with a Mallory–Weiss tear require:
    a Injection of adrenaline.
    b Endoscopic band ligation.
    c No therapeutic intervention.
    d Heater probe application.

56. A 65-year-old male patient is admitted to a cardiac intensive care unit following cardiac bypass surgery. Three days post-operatively he starts complaining of pain in the right upper quadrant of the abdomen. On clinical examination, there is tenderness in the right hypochondrium with a positive Murphy's sign. His liver function test shows an ALT of 85 IU/L, normal bilirubin and alkaline phosphatase. Ultrasound shows a thick gallbladder wall with peri-cholecystic fluid but no calculi. The treatment of choice is:
    a Emergency laparoscopic cholecystectomy.
    b Antibiotics and interval cholecystectomy.
    c Percutaneous cholecystostomy and antibiotics.
    d No further treatment.

57. All of the following statements with regard to the pathophysiology of cholangitis are false, except:
    a It results when there is biliary obstruction and infection.
    b Obstruction or infection alone does not result in cholangitis.
    c 50% of patients with cholangitis present with shock.
    d The majority of patients present with abdominal pain, jaundice and fever.

58. The preferred treatment of choice in an elderly patient with a significant cardiac history and acute cholecystitis not responding to medical treatment is:
   a Emergency cholecystectomy.
   b Percutaneous cholecystostomy.
   c Endoscopic retrograde cholangiopancreatography (ERCP) and sphincterotomy.
   d Open cholecystostomy.

59. The ideal time for cholecystectomy in patients with mild gallstone pancreatitis is:
   a <48 hours following admission.
   b Within 6 weeks following discharge from hospital.
   c During the same admission.
   d After complete resolution of symptoms.

60. The most common cause of small bowel obstruction is:
   a Inguinal hernia.
   b Adhesions.
   c Malignancy.
   d Umbilical hernia.

61. Richter's hernia is:
   a Incarceration of part of the circumference of the bowel.
   b Inguinal hernia with both a direct and indirect hernia component.
   c Presence of the appendix in the hernial sac.
   d Hernia through the arcuate line.

62. The recommended maximum dose of lignocaine as a local anaesthetic is:
   a 2 mg/kg.
   b 3 mg/kg.
   c 1 mg/kg.
   d 7 mg/kg.

63. The most likely diagnosis in a 75-year-old female with a history of atrial fibrillation presenting with vague central abdominal pain and minimal abdominal signs is:
   a Acute small bowel obstruction.
   b Mesenteric ischaemia.
   c Diverticulitis.
   d Acute appendicitis.

64. A 25-year-old male presents with a 4-day history of right iliac fossa pain associated with nausea and anorexia. His pulse rate is 90/min and temperature 37.8°C. Abdominal examination reveals a mass in the right iliac fossa. His white cell count is 11,500/mm^3. The most appropriate management of this patient is:
   a Appendicectomy.
   b Laparotomy and limited ileocaecal resection.
   c Laparotomy and right hemicolectomy.
   d Conservative management and barium enema after a few weeks before considering for surgery.

65. All of the following are advantages of laparoscopic appendicectomy, except:
   a Less post-operative pain.
   b Early return to work.
   c Reduced hospital stay.
   d Lower incidence of intra-abdominal abscess.

66. The parts of the colon which are most vulnerable to ischaemia are:
   a Griffiths' point at the splenic flexure.
   b Mid-sigmoid colon at the junction of the inferior mesenteric artery and hypogastric vasculature.
   c Caecum.
   d All of the above.
   e None of the above.

67. An 85-year-old male patient with a previous history of ischaemic heart disease, diabetes and hypertension presents with sudden onset of severe bloody diarrhoea. The most likely cause of bloody diarrhoea is:
   a Ischaemic colitis.
   b Diverticular disease.
   c Rectal malignancy.
   d Duodenal ulcer.

68. The most common site of colonic volvulus is the:
   a Sigmoid colon.
   b Caecum.
   c Transverse colon.
   d Ileocaecal junction.

69. A 70-year-old male patient presents with a 4-day history of abdominal pain, associated with constipation and abdominal distension. There is no significant past medical history. On examination, there is marked asymmetrical abdominal distension and tympanitic note on percussion. The next most appropriate investigation of choice is:
   a Barium enema.
   b Gastrografin enema.
   c X-ray abdomen.
   d Computed tomography with rectal contrast.

70. The diagnostic investigation of choice in a patient with suspected sigmoid volvulus is:
   a Barium enema.
   b Gastrografin enema.
   c X-ray abdomen.
   d Computed tomography with rectal contrast.

71. The amount of bleeding necessary to be identified by a Technetium-99 tacked red blood cell scan is:
   a 0.1–0.5 mL/min.
   b 1–1.5 mL/min.
   c 2–3 mL/min.
   d Less than 0.1 mL/min.

72. The amount of bleeding that is necessary to be identified by angiography is:
   a 0.1–0.5 mL/min.
   b 1–1.5 mL/min.
   c 2–3 mL/min.
   d Less than 0.1 mL/min.

73. A 45-year-old male patient presents with severe bleeding per rectum. On examination his pulse rate is 120/min and BP 80/60 mmHg. His haemoglobin is 8.5 gm%. The most appropriate initial investigation of choice is:
   a Mesenteric angiography.
   b Colonoscopy.
   c Computed tomographic angiography.
   d Upper gastrointestinal endoscopy.

74. The diagnostic investigation of choice for the confirmation of Hirschsprung's disease is:
    a Water soluble contrast enema.
    b Rectal biopsy.
    c Transanal ultrasound.
    d Anorectal manometry.

75. The most likely diagnosis in a 4-week-old baby boy with projectile vomiting after feeding and a palpable mass in the epigastric region is:
    a Meconium ileus.
    b Small bowel intussusception.
    c Hypertrophic pyloric stenosis.
    d Obstructed inguinal hernia.

76. The electrolyte abnormalities associated with gastric outlet obstruction are:
    a Hypokalaemia, hyponatraemia, hyperchloraemia.
    b Hypokalaemia, hypernatraemia, hyperchloraemia.
    c Hyperkalaemia, hyponatraemia, hypochloraemia.
    d Hypokalaemia, hyponatraemia, hypochloraemia.

77. The metabolic abnormalities associated with gastric outlet obstruction are:
    a Metabolic acidosis with paradoxical alkaluria.
    b Metabolic alkalosis with paradoxical aciduria.
    c Respiratory alkalosis with compensated metabolic acidosis.
    d Respiratory acidosis with compensated metabolic alkalosis.

78. The investigation of choice in a child with suspected intussusception is:
    a CT of abdomen.
    b Ultrasound.
    c Colonoscopy.
    d X-ray of abdomen.

79. Which one of the following statements with regard to intussusception in children is incorrect?
   a Ileocolic intussusception is the most common type.
   b The majority of children with ileocolic intussusception present with intermittent abdominal pain, palpable mass and 'redcurrant jelly' stools.
   c Pneumatic reduction with air or carbon dioxide is associated with an 80–95% success rate.
   d The peak incidence is seen among the 6–9 month age group.

80. Surgical intervention is indicated in which of the following group of patients with intussusception:
   a Patients who failed hydrostatic or pneumatic reduction.
   b Patients with no signs of peritonitis.
   c Patients with no free gas on X-ray.
   d All of the above.

81. Bilious vomiting in neonates and children is usually due to:
   a Viral gastroenteritis.
   b Upper respiratory tract infection.
   c Appendicitis.
   d Intestinal obstruction.

82. The earliest sign of intravascular fluid depletion in children is:
   a Tachycardia.
   b Hypotension.
   c Low urine output.
   d Irritability.

83. A 15 kg, 4-year-old child presents with a 2-day history of vomiting and diarrhoea. On examination he is dehydrated with a pulse rate of 160/min. The most appropriate amount of fluid to resuscitate this child is:
   a 20 mL/kg bolus until signs of cardiovascular improvement.
   b 10 mL/kg bolus followed by 2 mL/kg maintenance fluid.
   c 4 mL/kg bolus followed by 2 mL/kg maintenance fluid.
   d 100 mL/kg bolus until signs of cardiovascular improvement.

84. The most likely diagnosis in a neonate who has not passed the meconium within 24 hours after birth is:
    a Hirschsprung's disease.
    b Anorectal malformation.
    c Meconium ileus.
    d Small bowel atresia.

85. The disadvantages of diagnostic peritoneal lavage (DPL) include all of the following, except:
    a It does not identify the organ of injury.
    b Retroperitoneal injuries can be missed.
    c Pelvic fracture can give false positive results.
    d It can be carried out in A&E.

86. Which one of the following statements with regard to a positive diagnostic peritoneal lavage (DPL) is incorrect?
    a Red cell count <100,000/mm^3.
    b White cell count >500/mm^3.
    c Presence of amylase.
    d Presence of bowel contents in DPL fluid.

87. A 30-year-old male driver is brought into A&E following a head-on collision with another car. At the time of arrival, his blood pressure is 80 mmHg, pulse rate 100/min and respiratory rate 28/min. On examination, there is mild tenderness over the lower chest and generalised abdominal tenderness particularly over the right upper abdomen. Chest X-ray reveals 10th and 11th rib fractures. Pelvic X-ray shows fracture of both pubic rami. There is no improvement in his vital signs despite fluid resuscitation. Focused abdominal sonography for trauma (FAST) scan shows a large amount of fluid in the Morrison pouch. The management of this patient includes:
    a Laparotomy.
    b Pelvic angiography and embolisation of bleeding vessels.
    c Stabilisation of the pelvis followed by laparotomy.
    d Laparotomy followed by pelvic stabilisation.

88. Abdominal compartment syndrome is defined as a sustained intra-abdominal pressure of more than:
    a 20 mmHg.
    b 15 mmH$_2$O.
    c 45 mmHg.
    d 12 mmHg.

89. All of the following changes are associated with raised intra-abdominal pressure, except:
    a Decreased central venous pressure.
    b Increased airway pressure.
    c Reduction in tidal volume.
    d Decreased renal output.

90. Raised intra-abdominal pressure is associated with all of the following changes in cardiac function, except:
    a Decreased cardiac output.
    b Increased central venous pressure.
    c Increased preload.
    d Decreased stroke volume.

91. Increased intra-abdominal pressure is associated with all of the following changes in respiratory function, except:
    a Increased lung compliance.
    b Increased airway pressure.
    c Diaphragmatic splinting.
    d Reduction in tidal volume.

92. The most common cause of a venous thromboembolism is:
    a Idiopathic.
    b Malignancy.
    c Anti-phospholipid syndrome.
    d Recent surgery.

93. Which one of the following statements with regard to the natural history of venous thromboembolism (VTE) is incorrect?
    a Most deep vein thrombosis (DVT) starts in the calf veins.
    b The risk of VTE is highest within 2 weeks following surgery.
    c Isolated calf DVTs are rarely symptomatic.
    d The greatest risk of post-operative pulmonary embolism is within 48 hours after surgery.

94. Protein C is synthesised in the:
    a Liver.
    b Megakaryocytes.
    c Endothelial cells.
    d Leukocytes.

95. The half-life of prothrombin is:
a   6 hours.
b   36 hours.
c   48 hours.
d   72 hours.

96. Which one of the following statements with regard to heparin-induced thrombocytopenia (HIT) is incorrect?
a   Unfractionated heparin is associated with a higher incidence of HIT compared to low molecular weight heparin.
b   Patients receiving therapeutic treatment are at high risk compared to those receiving prophylactic treatment.
c   Medical patients are at high risk compared to surgical patients.
d   It is due to antibodies against platelet factor IV.

97. The most prevalent genetic risk factor for venous thromboembolism in the Caucasian population is:
a   Factor V Leiden deficiency.
b   Anti-phospholipid syndrome.
c   Homocysteinemia.
d   Anti-thrombin deficiency.

98. Anti-phospholipid syndrome is due to:
a   Anti-cardiolipin antibodies.
b   Protein C deficiency.
c   Anti-thrombin deficiency.
d   Elevated factor III levels.

99. All of the following are side-effects of heparin, except:
a   Thrombocytopenia.
b   Hypokalaemia.
c   Osteoporosis.
d   Alopecia.

100. Which one of the following statements with regard to heparin-induced thrombocytopenia (HIT) is incorrect?
a Heparin should be stopped and the patient started on alternative anticoagulants.
b Warfarin should not be started until the platelet count is fully recovered.
c Prophylactic platelet transfusion should be given due to the risk of bleeding.
d None of the above.

101. A 60-year-old female presents with a sudden onset of left lower leg pain associated with swelling and erythema. The most likely diagnosis is:
a Osteoarthritis of left knee.
b Deep vein thrombosis.
c Acute popliteal artery thrombosis.
d Ruptured Baker's cyst.

102. A 35-year-old female presents with a sudden onset of painful swollen white leg. There is no significant past medical history. The most likely diagnosis is:
a Femoral artery embolism.
b Femoral vein thrombosis.
c Thrombosis of both iliac veins.
d Ruptured Baker's cyst.

103. The gold standard test for the diagnosis of deep vein thrombosis is:
a Doppler ultrasound.
b Venography.
c Magnetic resonance angiography.
d Impedance plethysmography.

104. The investigation of choice for the diagnosis of deep vein thrombosis is:
a Doppler ultrasound.
b Venography.
c Magnetic resonance angiography.
d Impedance plethysmography.

105. A 35-year-old female with a history of systemic lupus erythema-
tosis (SLE) presents with a 2-day history of right-sided chest pain
and shortness of breath. Clinical examination reveals a right-sided
pleural rub with good and equal air entry on both sides. ECG shows
sinus tachycardia. Chest X-ray is unremarkable. The most likely
diagnosis is:
   a Pulmonary embolism.
   b Pneumonia.
   c Right-sided heart failure.
   d Acute cholecystitis.

106. The predominant mode of action of low molecular weight heparin
is:
   a Inhibition of factor Xa.
   b Inhibition of factor IIa.
   c Inhibition of factor Va.
   d Inhibition of factor IXa.

107. The treatment of choice for deep vein thrombosis during pregnancy
is:
   a Warfarin.
   b Low molecular weight heparin.
   c Danaparoid.
   d Fondaparinux.

108. Which one of the following statements with regard to fondaparinux
is incorrect?
   a It is a selective inhibitor of factor Xa.
   b It is a pentasaccharide.
   c Once daily dose is as effective as low molecular weight heparin.
   d It can cause thrombocytopenia.

109. Which one of the following vitamin K dependent clotting factors
has a half-life of 6 hours?
   a Factor II.
   b Factor VII.
   c Factor IX.
   d Factor X.

110. The advantages of low molecular weight heparin compared to unfractionated heparin include all of the following, except:
    a Fewer bleeding complications.
    b It has a longer biological half-life.
    c Levels do not require regular monitoring.
    d It is associated with a lower incidence of type II heparin-induced thrombocytopenia (HIT).

111. The risk factors for re-feeding syndrome include all, except:
    a Hypokalaemia.
    b Hypomagnesaemia.
    c Hypophosphataemia.
    d Renal failure.

112. Which one of the following statements with regard to re-feeding syndrome is incorrect?
    a Patients with hypokalaemia, hypomagnesaemia and hypophosphataemia are at high risk.
    b Re-feeding syndrome can give rise to life-threatening cardiac arrhythmias.
    c Thiamine deficiency is the most common vitamin deficiency associated with re-feeding syndrome.
    d Patients at high risk of developing re-feeding syndrome should be started with full calorie and protein requirements on the first day.

113. All of the following measures are part of peri-operative goal directed therapy, except:
    a Increased intravenous fluids using flow directed monitoring equipment to maximise intravascular filling pressure.
    b Maintenance of adequate haemoglobulin concentration.
    c Maintenance of 100% oxygenation saturation with supplemental oxygenation.
    d Maintenance of mean arterial pressure of 60 mmHg by non-adrenaline infusion.

114. Which one of the following agents is very effective in improving cardiac index and oxygen delivery:
    a Adrenaline.
    b Dobutamine.
    c Noradrenaline.
    d Dopexamine.

115. Cryoprecipitate contains all of the following factors, except:
   a Fibrinogen.
   b Anti-thrombin.
   c von Willebrand factor (VWF).
   d Factor VIII.

116. The ebb phase of stress response is associated with which one of the following changes:
   a Increased resting energy expenditure.
   b Increased glucose intolerance.
   c Increased glycogenolysis.
   d Increased gluconeogenesis.

117. Glucose is the main source of energy for which of the following structures:
   a Leukocytes, red blood cells (RBC), brain.
   b Leukocytes, RBC, brain, kidney.
   c Muscle, RBC, leukocyte, brain.
   d Brain, epithelial cell, leukocyte, muscle.

118. C-reactive protein is synthesised in the:
   a Leukocyte.
   b Lung.
   c Liver.
   d Small bowel.

119. Which of the following parameters are used as part of a malnutrition universal screening tool (MUST) in the assessment of the risk of malnutrition?
   a Body mass index (BMI).
   b Percentage of unplanned weight loss in 3–6 months.
   c Illness of the patient.
   d All of the above.

120. The contraindications for enteral nutritional support include all of the following, except:
   a Small bowel obstruction.
   b Vomiting and diarrhoea.
   c High output intestinal fistula.
   d Cerebrovascular accident.

121. A 40-year-old male patient develops hypotension following central line insertion for nutritional support. Respiratory examination is unremarkable. Cardiovascular examination reveals a machinery murmur over the mediastinum. Chest X-ray does not show any evidence of widening of the mediastinum, tracheal deviation or collapsed lung. The most likely diagnosis is:
    a Pneumothorax.
    b Air embolism.
    c Haemopneumothorax.
    d Mediastinal haematoma.

122. The most common complication associated with central line insertion is:
    a Central line infection.
    b Thrombosis of central vein.
    c Pneumothorax.
    d Haemothorax.

123. Damage to which of the following nerves results in inguinal hernia formation following appendicectomy:
    a Iliohypogastric nerve.
    b Genital branch of the genitofemoral nerve.
    c Lateral cutaneous nerve of the thigh.
    d Ilioinguinal nerve.

124. All of the following arteries originate from the ventral aspect of the abdominal aorta, except the:
    a Coeliac artery.
    b Superior mesenteric artery.
    c Inferior mesenteric artery.
    d Lumbar artery.

125. The medial boundary of the ischiorectal fossa is formed by the:
    a Urogenital diaphragm.
    b Fascia covering the levator ani muscle.
    c Sacrotuberous ligament and gluteus maximus.
    d Fascia covering the obturator internus and ischeal tuberosity.

126. All of the following are the contents of Alcock's canal, except the:
    a Internal pudendal vessel.
    b Pudendal nerve.
    c Inferior rectal branch of the internal pudendal artery.
    d Nerve to the obturator internus.

127. The root supply of the pudendal nerve is:
    a L4, 5, S1.
    b S 2, 3, 4.
    c S 1, 2, 3.
    d L5, S1, 2.

128. The external anal sphincter is supplied by the:
    a Inferior rectal nerve.
    b Ileoinguinal nerve.
    c Genital branch of the genitofemoral nerve.
    d Iliohypogastric nerve.

129. Which of the following nutrients are absorbed via the lymphatics?
    a Long-chain fatty acids.
    b Medium-chain fatty acids.
    c Short-chain fatty acids.
    d Medium- and short-chain fatty acids.

130. The umbilical vein carries:
    a Purified blood from the placenta to the liver through the left branch of the portal vein.
    b Purified blood from the inferior vena cava through the portal vein.
    c Unpurified blood from the liver to the placenta.
    d Purified blood from the placenta to the liver through the right branch of the portal vein.

131. The reason for referred pain to the skin overlying the right acromian process in patients with acute cholecystitis is:
    a The phrenic nerve arises from the same segment of spinal cord as the supraclavicular nerves.
    b The gallbladder is innervated by the supraclavicular nerves.
    c The gallbladder develops from the foregut.
    d The liver capsule, innervated by the phrenic nerve, is stretched.

132. All of the following are boundaries of Morrison's pouch, except the:
   a Superior surface of the liver.
   b Peritoneum covering the diaphragm and upper pole of the right kidney.
   c Coronary ligament.
   d None of the above.

133. The anterior border of the foramen of Winslow is formed by the:
   a Inferior vena cava and right adrenal gland.
   b Caudate lobe of liver.
   c Right free border of the lesser omentum.
   d First part of the duodenum.

134. The lienorenal ligament contains:
   a Short gastric vessels.
   b Tail of the pancreas.
   c Left gastric artery.
   d Left renal vein.

135. Which one of the following statements regarding the blood supply to the spleen is incorrect?
   a The splenic artery arises from the coeliac artery.
   b The intrasplenic branches of the splenic artery usually do not anastomose with each other.
   c The segmental blood supply makes segmental splenic resection possible.
   d Anterior and posterior segments have their own blood supply separated by an avascular plane.

136. The most common site of an undescended testis is the:
   a Inguinal canal.
   b Lumbar region.
   c Iliac region.
   d Renal angle.

137. Varicocoele is more common on the left side due to:
   a Absence of valves on the left side.
   b Long left renal vein.
   c Left testicular vein entering the renal vein at a right angle.
   d None of the above.

138. The angle of Louis corresponds to all of the following, except:
   a Bifurcation of the trachea.
   b Lower border of the 2nd thoracic vertebra.
   c Meeting point of both mediastinal pleura.
   d The beginning of the ascent of the arch of the aorta.

139. The segment of the right lung that is frequently affected by aspiration pneumonia is the:
   a Lateral basal segment of the lower lobe.
   b Apical segment of the right upper lobe.
   c Posterior segment of the right upper lobe.
   d Medial segment of the middle lobe.

140. Which of the following group of patients are at high risk of airway compromise?
   a Unconscious patients with head injuries.
   b Patients with a history of alcohol intake.
   c Patients with thoracic injuries.
   d All of the above.

141. A 35-year-old male driver was brought to A&E following a road traffic accident. On arrival to A&E his Glasgow Coma Score is 15/15. However, he is suspected to have laryngeal trauma. Which of the following signs indicate the presence of laryngeal trauma?
   a Hoarseness.
   b Subcutaneous emphysema.
   c Palpable fracture of the larynx.
   d All of the above.

142. The relative contraindications for nasotracheal intubation include:
   a Bilateral ecchymosis of the periorbital region.
   b Presence of post-auricular ecchymosis.
   c Presence of cerebrospinal fluid (CSF) otorrhea.
   d All of the above.

143. The main intracellular buffer system is:
   a Bicarbonate.
   b Phosphate.
   c Plasma proteins.
   d Cytoplasmic proteins.

144. The normal base deficit is:
a −2 to +2.
b −5 to +5.
c −10 to +10.
d −1 to +1.

145. Noradrenaline does not cause:
a Increased heart rate.
b Increased stroke volume.
c Increased mean arterial pressure.
d Vasoconstriction.

146. Dopamine does not cause:
a Increased heart rate.
b Decreased stroke volume.
c Increased mean arterial pressure.
d Vasoconstriction.

147. The ionotrope of choice in patients with suspected low cardiac output in the presence of adequate left ventricular filling pressure is:
a Dopamine.
b Dobutamine.
c Noradrenaline.
d Adrenaline.

148. Cryoprecipitate is rich in:
a Factor VIII.
b Factor II.
c Factor XII.
d Factor X.

149. The half-life of neutrophils is:
a 6 hours.
b 12 hours.
c 24 hours.
d 1 week.

150. The half-life of platelets is:
a 6 hours.
b 4 days.
c 1 week.
d 24 hours.

151. The normal oncotic pressure across capillary walls is:
   a 25 mmHg.
   b 12 mmHg.
   c 5 mmHg.
   d 10 mmHg.

152. The extrinsic clotting pathway is activated by:
   a Tissue thromboplastin.
   b Factor Xa.
   c Factor XIIa.
   d Factor Va.

153. Which one of the following is not a vitamin K dependent clotting factor?
   a Factor II.
   b Factor V.
   c Factor VII.
   d Factor XII.

154. Fresh frozen plasma is normally stored at:
   a −40 to −50°C.
   b 4°C.
   c −4°C.
   d 0°C.

155. The majority of CO_2 is transported in the blood in the following form:
   a Bicarbonate ions.
   b Carbamino compounds.
   c Physically dissolved in solution.
   d Bound to haemoglobin.

156. The shape of the CO_2 dissociation curve is:
   a Sigmoid.
   b Curvilinear.
   c Linear.
   d Hyperbolic.

157. The Bohr effect describes:
    a The affinity of haemoglobin for O_2 following variation in $paCO_2$, H^+ ion and temperature.
    b The affinity of blood for CO_2 and variations in $paCO_2$.
    c The relationship between chloride ion and bicarbonate effect in the red blood cell.
    d The relationship between H^+ and Cl^- inside the red blood cell.

158. All of the following are functions of the colon, except:
    a Absorption of sodium ions.
    b Absorption of water.
    c Absorption of potassium and bicarbonate ions.
    d Synthesis of vitamin K.

159. The coronary artery originates from the:
    a Ascending aorta just above the aortic valve leaflets.
    b Ascending aorta just below the aortic valve leaflets.
    c Arch of aorta proximal to the ductus arteriosus.
    d Arch of aorta distal to the ductus arteriosus.

160. Coronary blood flow is at its maximum during which part of the cardiac cycle:
    a Diastole.
    b Systole.
    c Both systole and diastole.
    d Isovolumetric contraction.

161. The most common site of oesophageal perforation in Boerhaave's syndrome is the:
    a Cervical oesophagus.
    b Upper third of the thoracic oesophagus.
    c Middle third of the thoracic oesophagus.
    d Lower third of the thoracic oesophagus.

162. All of the following criteria are used in the modified Glasgow scale severity scoring system for pancreatitis, except:
    a Serum calcium.
    b Serum albumin.
    c LDH.
    d Temperature.

163. The most common cause of decreased levels of consciousness in a general surgical patient is:
    a Hypoxia.
    b Hypovolaemia.
    c Sepsis.
    d Analgesics.

164. All of the following conditions can cause respiratory failure due to an acute fall in functional residual capacity, except:
    a Chest trauma.
    b Post-operative atelectasis.
    c Respiratory depression due to analgesics.
    d Left ventricular failure.

165. Pulse oximeters do not detect:
    a Hypercapnia.
    b Acidosis.
    c Hypoxia.
    d a and b.

166. The fractional inspired oxygen concentration of atmospheric air is:
    a 0.6.
    b 0.2.
    c 0.1.
    d 0.4.

167. A SaO_2 of 90% often equates with a PaO_2 of:
    a 90 mmHg.
    b 60 mmHg.
    c 50 mmHg.
    d 100 mmHg.

168. The type of haemoglobin that can give an erroneous high reading on a pulse oximeter is:
    a Oxyhaemoglobin.
    b Carboxyhaemoglobin.
    c Methaemoglobin.
    d Sickle cell haemoglobin.

169. Which one of the following conditions does not produce mediastinal shift?
    a Collapse of lung.
    b Haemothorax.
    c Pneumothorax.
    d Consolidation.

170. Kerley B lines are caused by:
    a Increased fluid within the intralobular septa of the lung.
    b Increased tissue within the intralobular septa of the lung.
    c Both of the above.
    d None of the above.

171. In blast injury, which of the following organs is least vulnerable to the blast wave?
    a Small bowel.
    b Lungs.
    c Liver.
    d Ear drum.

172. A 15-year-old boy presents to A&E following a road traffic accident with left upper quadrant pain. On clinical examination, his pulse rate is 100/min, blood pressure 110/60 mmHg and tenderness over the left 9th and 10th ribs. Chest X-ray shows fractures of the 9th, 10th and 11th ribs. An urgent CT abdomen shows free fluid around the spleen and splenic laceration with no leakage of contrast. The most appropriate treatment is:
    a Observation.
    b Splenectomy.
    c Arterial embolisation.
    d Splenorrhaphy.

173. The most common organ injured in a penetrating abdominal injury is the:
    a Liver.
    b Spleen.
    c Colon.
    d Small bowel.

174. Platelets can be stored at:
a 20–24°C for 5 days.
b 20–24°C for 8 days.
c 4–8°C for 5 days.
d 4–8°C for 8 days.

175. All of the following are electrocardiographic features of hyperkalaemia, except:
a Prolonged PR interval.
b Prolonged QT interval.
c Sine wave patterns.
d Loss of P waves.

176. Hypochloraemia, hypokalaemia and metabolic alkalosis are seen in:
a Congenital hypertrophic pyloric stenosis.
b Hirschsprung's disease.
c Oesophageal atresia.
d Jejunal atresia.

177. Persistent vomiting can cause all of the following, except:
a Hypokalaemia.
b Decreased K^+ in the urine.
c Elevated blood pH.
d Metabolic alkalosis.

178. Complications of massive blood transfusion include all, except:
a Hypokalaemia.
b Hypothermia.
c Hypomagnesaemia.
d Hypocalcaemia.

179. The normal range of serum osmolality (in mOsm/L) is:
a 270 to 285.
b 300 to 320.
c 350 to 375.
d 200 to 250.

180. All of the following infections may be transmitted via blood transfusion, except:
    a Parvovirus.
    b Dengue virus.
    c Cytomegalovirus (CMV).
    d Hepatitis G virus.

181. Measurement of intravascular pressure with a pulmonary artery catheter should be done:
    a At the end of expiration.
    b At the peak of inspiration.
    c During mid-inspiration.
    d During mid-expiration.

182. A 70-year-old female being treated with antibiotics for acute cholecystitis develops increased pain and tenderness in the right upper quadrant with a palpable mass. She develops hematemesis, melena and a petechial rash with a temperature increase to 40°C (104°F) and blood pressure reduction to 80/60 mmHg. Laboratory studies reveal thrombocytopenia, prolonged prothrombin time and decreased fibrinogen level. The most important step in the correction of this patient's coagulopathy is:
    a Exploratory laparotomy.
    b Administration of heparin.
    c Administration of e-aminocaproic acid.
    d Administration of fresh frozen plasma.

183. Which one of the following complications is most likely following a massive blood transfusion?
    a Metabolic alkalosis.
    b Metabolic acidosis.
    c Respiratory alkalosis.
    d Respiratory acidosis.

184. The most common route of transmission of hepatitis E is:
    a Blood transfusion.
    b Faeco-oral.
    c Intercourse.
    d Intravenous injection.

185. The deep inguinal ring is a defect in the:
      a Internal oblique muscle.
      b Transversus abdominis muscle.
      c Internal spermatic fascia.
      d Transversalis fascia.

186. Injury to which of the following nerves during inguinal hernia repair
      can give rise to anaesthesia at the root of the penis and adjacent part
      of the scrotum?
      a Genital branch of the genitofemoral nerve.
      b Femoral branch of the genitofemoral nerve.
      c Iliohypogastric nerve.
      d Ilioinguinal nerve.

187. The primary treatment modality of choice for desmoid tumour is:
      a Surgery.
      b Chemotherapy.
      c Radiotherapy.
      d Surgery and radiotherapy.

188. The most common content in 'hernia-en-glissade' is the:
      a Omentum.
      b Urinary bladder.
      c Caecum.
      d Sigmoid colon.

189. The most common sliding component of a direct hernia is the:
      a Bladder.
      b Caecum.
      c Ascending colon.
      d Descending colon.

190. The most common hernia to strangulate is:
      a Direct inguinal hernia.
      b Indirect inguinal hernia.
      c Femoral hernia.
      d Epigastric hernia.

191. Foreign body aspiration in a supine position commonly affects which of the following parts of the lung?
    a Left apical lobe.
    b Right apical lobe.
    c Apical part of the right lower lobe.
    d Postero-basal segment of the left lung.

192. The most common cause of death in penetrating injury to the chest is:
    a Chylothorax.
    b Pulmonary contusion.
    c Tracheobronchial injury.
    d Oesophageal rupture.

193. The treatment of choice in severe flail chest is:
    a Strapping.
    b Intercostal nerve block.
    c Fixation of the fractured ribs with wire.
    d Intermittent positive pressure ventilation (IPPV).

194. Which of the following muscles is not cut during a postero-lateral thoracotomy?
    a Serratus anterior.
    b Latissimus dorsi.
    c Rhomboid major.
    d Pectoralis major.

195. The first-line treatment for a keloid is:
    a Intralesional injection of steroid.
    b Local steroid application.
    c Radiotherapy.
    d Wide excision.

196. The most common site of keloid is the:
    a Face.
    b Leg.
    c Presternal area.
    d Arm.

197. Marjolin's ulcer is a:
 a Malignant ulcer found on the scar of a burn.
 b Malignant ulcer found on an infected foot.
 c Trophic ulcer.
 d Meleney's gangrene.

198. Which one of the following statements about keloids is correct?
 a They are more common in white people than in black people.
 b They do not extend into normal skin.
 c Local recurrence is common after excision.
 d They frequently undergo malignant change.

199. The most common retroperitoneal tumour is:
 a Fibrosarcoma.
 b Liposarcoma.
 c Dermoid cyst.
 d Rhabdomyosarcoma.

200. Which one of the following soft tissue sarcomas frequently metastasises to lymph nodes?
 a Fibrosarcoma.
 b Osteosarcoma.
 c Embryonal rhabdomyosarcoma.
 d Liposarcoma.

201. During which phase of the cell cycle is the cellular DNA content doubled?
 a Mitotic phase.
 b G1 phase.
 c G2 phase.
 d S phase.

202. The tumour suppressor gene p^{53} induces cell cycle arrest at:
 a G_2– M phase.
 b S–G_2 phase.
 c G_1–S phase.
 d G_0 phase.

203. Programmed cell death is known as:
  a Cytolysis.
  b Apoptosis.
  c Necrosis.
  d Proptosis.

204. α-fetoprotein is elevated in which of the following tumours?
  a Choriocarcinoma.
  b Neuroblastoma.
  c Hepatocellular carcinoma.
  d Seminoma.

205. Which of the following radioactive isotopes is not used for brachytherapy?
  a Iodine-125.
  b Iodine-131.
  c Cobalt-60.
  d Iridium-192.

206. Women receiving oestrogen therapy have an increased risk of developing all of the following cancers, except:
  a Breast cancer.
  b Endometrial carcinoma.
  c Carcinoma of the gallbladder.
  d Hepatocellular carcinoma.

207. Epstein–Barr virus is associated with:
  a Carcinoma of the larynx.
  b Carcinoma of the urinary bladder.
  c Carcinoma of the nasopharynx.
  d Carcinoma of the maxilla.

208. In computed tomography (CT), the attenuation values are measured in Hounsfield units (HU). An attenuation value of 0 (zero) HU corresponds to:
  a Water.
  b Air.
  c Very dense bone structure.
  d Fat.

209. Which of the following diagnostic investigations uses piezoelectric crystals?
   a Ultrasonography.
   b Nuclear magnetic resonance (NMR) imaging.
   c X-ray diffraction.
   d Xeroradiography.

210. Radiation therapy to hypoxic tissues may be potentiated by treatment with:
   a Mycostatin.
   b Metronidazole.
   c Methotrexate.
   d Melphalan.

211. Transition from G2 to M phase of the cell cycle is controlled by:
   a Retinoblastoma gene product.
   b p53 protein.
   c Cyclin E.
   d Cyclin B.

212. Tumour lysis syndrome is associated with all of the following laboratory features, except:
   a Hyperkalaemia.
   b Hypercalcaemia.
   c Hyperuricaemia.
   d Hyperphosphataemia.

213. The drug of choice for cisplatin-induced emesis is:
   a Metoclopramide.
   b Domperidone.
   c Ondansetron.
   d Octreotide.

214. The tissue most sensitive to radiation is the:
   a Skin.
   b Liver.
   c Ovary.
   d Spleen.

215. Hypercalcaemia associated with malignancy is most often mediated by:
  a Parathyroid hormone (PTH).
  b Parathyroid hormone related protein (PTHrP).
  c Interleukin-6 (IL-6).
  d Calcitonin.

216. Which of the following radio-isotopes is commonly used as a source for external beam radiotherapy in the treatment of cancer patients?
  a Strontium-89.
  b Radium-226.
  c Cobalt-59.
  d Cobalt-60.

217. The phase of cell cycle that is most sensitive to radiotherapy is:
  a S_2 phase.
  b G_1 phase.
  c G_2 phase.
  d G_2–M phase.

218. Which of the following tumours are not radio-responsive?
  a Hodgkin's lymphoma.
  b Malignant melanoma.
  c Ewing's sarcoma.
  d Seminoma.

219. Ototoxicity and nephrotoxicity are frequently encountered following therapy with which of the following:
  a Bleomycin.
  b Cyclophosphamide.
  c Cisplatinium.
  d 5-fluorouracil.

220. The intra-abdominal pressure during laparoscopy should be set between:
  a 5–8 mmHg.
  b 10–14 mmHg.
  c 20–25 mmHg.
  d 30–35 mmHg.

221. The following gas is used to create pneumoperitoneum in laparoscopy:
    a CO_2.
    b N_2O.
    c O_2.
    d N_2.

222. The survival of skin grafts within 48 hours following transplantation depends on:
    a The amount of saline in the graft.
    b Plasma imbibition.
    c The new vessels growing from the donor tissue.
    d The connection between the donor and recipient capillaries.

223. Which one of the following statements regarding skin grafting is incorrect?
    a Partial thickness grafts include the epidermis and part of the dermis.
    b Full thickness grafts include the epidermis and dermis.
    c Full thickness grafts are mainly used for large areas of defect.
    d Full thickness grafts result in better cosmetic appearance than split thickness skin grafts.

224. Which one of the following changes is not associated with deep burns?
    a Hyperthermia.
    b Increased vascular permeability.
    c Fluid loss by evaporation.
    d Vasodilatation.

225. The treatment of choice for Dupuytren's contracture is:
    a Passive stretching.
    b Hydrocortisone infiltration.
    c Total fasciectomy.
    d Subcutaneous fasciectomy.

226. For re-implantation surgery, the detached digit or limb is best preserved in:
    a Ice packs.
    b Distilled water.
    c Hypertonic saline.
    d Isotonic saline.

227. Deep burns are associated with all of the following characteristics, except:
    a Loss of pain sensation.
    b Charred appearance.
    c Loss of skin reaction.
    d Presence of blisters.

228. The most effective fluid for resuscitation of burns patients is:
    a Lactated Ringer's solution.
    b Hexaethyl starch.
    c 5% dextrose.
    d Blood.

229. The percentage area of burn in a child aged one year with burns to the head, face and neck is:
    a 18%.
    b 13%.
    c 9%.
    d 5%.

230. A graft from a different species is called:
    a Homograft.
    b Heterograft.
    c Xenograft.
    d Isograft.

231. The 'rule of nine' (Wallace) is used to calculate the percentage of the body surface area involved in a burns patient. Involvement of the head and neck together constitutes:
    a 1%.
    b 7%.
    c 9%.
    d 18%.

232. The severity of burns with vesiculation, destruction of the epidermis and upper dermis are:
    a 1st degree.
    b 2nd degree.
    c 3rd degree.
    d 4th degree.

233. Radial nerve palsy causes:
    a Claw hand.
    b Wrist drop.
    c Policeman tip deformity.
    d Erb's palsy.

234. Post-burn contractures can be best prevented by:
    a Use of local antibiotics.
    b Early skin grafting.
    c Mafenamide application.
    d Silverex and mafenamide application.

235. The treatment of choice for a patient with a 4 cm retroperitoneal lymph node mass due to a non-seminomatous germ cell tumour of the testis is:
    a Radical radiotherapy.
    b High orchidectomy and retroperitoneal lymph node dissection.
    c Retroperitoneal lymph node dissection and chemotherapy.
    d High orchidectomy and chemotherapy.

236. Infertility is a common feature in Sertoli cell syndrome because:
    a Too many Sertoli cells inhibit spermatogenesis via inhibin.
    b A proper blood testis barrier is not established.
    c There are no germ cells.
    d Sufficient numbers of spermatozoa are not produced.

237. Which of the following statements regarding germ cell tumours of the testis is incorrect?
    a They constitute 90% of all primary testicular tumours.
    b Seminomas are the most common tumour to develop in patients with cryptorchidism.
    c α-fetoprotein is markedly raised in all germ cell tumours.
    d High inguinal orchidectomy is the initial surgical procedure of choice.

238. In patients with cryptorchidism, all of the following complications can be prevented by orchidopexy, except:
    a Testicular tumours.
    b Epididymo-orchitis.
    c Torsion of the testis.
    d Sexual ambiguity.

239. Which of the following statements regarding vaginal hydrocoele is true?
a It remains in the scrotum.
b It is confined to the spermatic cord.
c It is confined to the inguinal canal.
d It communicates with the peritoneal canal.

240. A unilateral undescended testis is ideally surgically corrected at around:
a 2 months of age.
b 6 months of age.
c 12 months of age.
d 24 months of age.

241. The most common malignant testicular neoplasm is:
a Teratoma.
b Seminoma.
c Choriocarcinoma.
d Lymphoma.

242. At 8 months the testes descend into the:
a Superficial inguinal ring.
b Inguinal canal.
c Scrotum.
d Deep inguinal ring.

243. The chemotherapeutic regimen used in the treatment of metastatic testicular carcinomas is:
a Bleomycin, etoposide, cisplatin.
b Vinblastine, etoposide, cisplatin.
c Doxorubicin, 5-fluorouracil, mercaptopurine.
d Methotrexate, 5-fluorouracil, vincristine.

244. Seminomas correspond to which one of the following ovarian tumours:
a Choriocarcinoma.
b Dysgerminoma.
c Granulosa cell tumour.
d Adenocarcinoma of the ovary.

245. The testicular lymphatic vessels drain to the:
a   Inguinal lymph nodes.
b   Para-aortic lymph nodes.
c   Mesenteric lymph nodes.
d   Pelvic lymph nodes.

246. All of the following are predisposing factors for the development of torsion of the testis, except:
a   Inversion of testis.
b   Epididymo-orchitis.
c   Long meso-orchium.
d   High investment of the tunica vaginalis.

247. The risk of wound infection in patients with clean contaminated wounds is:
a   1–2%.
b   <10%.
c   15–20%.
d   <40%.

248. Antiembolic (TED) stockings work by which of the following mechanisms:
a   Increasing the velocity of venous blood.
b   Increasing the velocity of arterial blood.
c   Reducing the accumulation of lactic acid.
d   None of the above.

249. Intermittent pneumatic compression reduces deep vein thrombosis (DVT) by:
a   10-fold.
b   20-fold.
c   3-fold.
d   5-fold.

250. The variable that is not used in the calculation of the nutritional risk index is:
a   Serum albumin.
b   The patient's current weight.
c   Serum transferrin.
d   The patient's normal weight.

251. Which of the following statements regarding undescended testis is incorrect?
    a It is more common on the right side.
    b It is unlikely to descend if it has not descended within a month of birth.
    c The risk of cancer reduces dramatically if it is corrected within six years.
    d In 10% of patients there is a family history of an undescended testis.

252. The most common type of testicular tumour is:
    a Teratoma.
    b Seminoma.
    c Sertoli cell tumours.
    d Leydig cell tumours.

253. The pro-kinetic mechanism of action of erythromycin is due to its function as:
    a Motilin receptor agonist in the gastrointestinal tract.
    b Dopamine receptor antagonist in the gastrointestinal tract.
    c Dopamine receptor agonist in the gastrointestinal tract.
    d Serotonin receptor antagonist in the gastrointestinal tract.

254. The pro-kinetic mechanism of metoclopramide is due to its function as:
    a Motilin receptor agonist in the gastrointestinal tract.
    b Dopamine receptor antagonist in the gastrointestinal tract.
    c Dopamine receptor agonist in the gastrointestinal tract.
    d Serotonin receptor antagonist in the gastrointestinal tract.

255. Which one of the following statements regarding the adverse effects of malnutrition is incorrect?
    a Malnutrition leads to impaired immune responses.
    b Malnutrition increases the risk of wound infection and anastomotic leak.
    c Malnutrition does not impair thermoregulation.
    d Malnutrition predisposes to pressure sores and thromboembolism.

256. Which one of the following statements regarding the prevalence of malnutrition in the UK is correct?
  a 40% of adults living in care homes have a body mass index (BMI) of less than 20 kg/m².
  b <5% of the general population living at home is underweight with a BMI of less than 20 kg/m².
  c 10% of adults with chronic lung and kidney disease living at home are underweight.
  d 10–60% of hospitalised patients are at risk of malnutrition in UK hospitals.
  e All of the above.

257. The indications for enteral tube feeding are:
  a Patients with oesophageal obstruction secondary to malignancy.
  b Patients with small bowel obstruction.
  c Patients with short gut syndrome.
  d None of the above.

258. Which of the following statements regarding gastrostomy tube feeding is incorrect?
  a Patients who are likely to require nutritional support for more than 4–6 weeks should be considered for gastrostomy tube feeding.
  b Gastrostomy tubes should be left in position for at least 2 weeks before considering removal.
  c Patients who are likely to require nutritional support for less than 4 weeks should be considered for gastrostomy.
  d Free air is visible in almost 40% of patients following percutaneous gastrostomy (PEG) tube insertions.

259. Which of the following statements regarding daily nutritional requirements is incorrect?
  a Daily energy requirements are 20–30 kcal/kg/day.
  b Daily fluid requirements are 30–35 mL/kg/day plus the replacement of additional losses.
  c Malnourished patients and patients at risk of malnutrition might need low volumes of feed to avoid re-feeding syndrome.
  d Daily protein requirements are 2.0–2.5 g/kg/day.

260. Which of the following statements regarding re-feeding syndrome is incorrect?
    a Re-feeding problems arise due to severe deficiency of micronutrients and electrolytes.
    b To avoid re-feeding problems, feed should be started at high volumes and reduced over a period of time.
    c Severely malnourished patients are at high risk of developing re-feeding problems.
    d Patients with low potassium, phosphate and magnesium prior to feeding are at high risk of developing re-feeding syndrome.

261. Which of the following statements regarding the laboratory monitoring of patients on nutritional support is incorrect?
    a Electrolytes should be checked daily until they are stable.
    b Calcium and albumin should be checked once before the beginning of nutritional support and then twice weekly.
    c Magnesium and phosphate should be checked three times a week until stable.
    d Folate and vitamin B12 levels should be checked every week.
    e Iron and ferritin levels should be checked once every month.

262. Total parenteral nutrition is indicated in all of the following conditions, except:
    a Patients with prolonged ileus following recent low anterior resection and abdominal sepsis following an anastomotic leak.
    b Patients with small bowel fistula due to Crohn's disease.
    c Patients with short gut syndrome.
    d In patients following a recent uneventful laparotomy for left hemicolectomy.

263. All the following complications are associated with enteral feeding, except:
    a Bloating.
    b Diarrhoea.
    c Cholestasis
    d Hypophosphataemia.

264. Ventilated patients requiring nutritional support should receive low carbohydrate and high fat ratio nutrition for which one of the following reasons:
    a High levels of carbohydrate increase CO_2 production.
    b High levels of carbohydrate increase water requirements.
    c High levels of carbohydrate delay recovery from surgery.
    d High levels of carbohydrate cause re-feeding syndrome.

265. Most commercial enteral feed contains:
    a 10 kcal/mL energy.
    b 1.0 kcal/mL energy.
    c 5 kcal/mL energy.
    d 0.5 kcal/mL energy.

266. Gastrostomy tube feeding is relatively contraindicated in:
    a Gastro-oesophageal reflux.
    b Previous gastric surgery.
    c Ascites.
    d Extensive gastric ulceration.
    e All of the above.

267. The most common skin tumour is:
    a Basal cell carcinoma.
    b Squamous cell carcinoma.
    c Malignant melanoma.
    d Mycosis fungoides.

268. Basal cell carcinoma can be differentiated from other skin cancers by the absence of:
    a Distant metastases.
    b Local invasion.
    c Rapid increase in size.
    d None of the above.

269. The ideal excision margin for a malignant melanoma of 3 mm thickness is:
    a 0.5 cm.
    b 2 cm.
    c 1 cm.
    d 3 cm.

270. The most commonly used donor site for skin grafting is the:
   a Lateral surface of the forearm.
   b Back of the gluteus maximus.
   c Lateral surface of the thigh.
   d Skin over anterior iliac spine.

271. The ideal length of the tibia that should be left behind during below-knee amputation is:
   a 25 cm.
   b 8 cm.
   c 10 cm.
   d 15 cm.

Answers: General and emergency surgery

1. a Noradrenaline.

2. b Tracheostomy.

3. a ↑ pH.

4. d All of the above.

5. b Peripheral vascular resistance.

6. c Cardiac tamponade.

7. c Hypotension without tachycardia.

8. a Haemorrhagic shock.

9. a 7% of body weight.

10. c 1,500–2,000 mL.

11. a Fully cross-matched blood.

12. b Urine output.

13. d Neurogenic shock.

14. b Anterio-medial surface of the proximal tibia.

15. d X-ray of the abdomen.

16. a Retrograde urethrogram.

17. c Chest X-ray.

18. c Capnography.

19. d a and b.

20. b Focused abdominal sonography for trauma (FAST) scan.

21. b Endotracheal intubation.

22. d ↓ cardiac output, ↑ preload, ↓ peripheral vascular resistance, ↑ afterload.

23. c Laryngeal mask.

24. b Endotracheal intubation.

25. a The majority are symptomatic.

26. b The majority require surgical repair.

27. d b and c.

28. d Diabetes.

29. b 1 cm above the pubic tubercle.

30. c Transversalis fascia.

31. a 1 cm above the midpoint between the pubic tubercle and the anterior superior iliac spine.

32. a External oblique aponeurosis and conjoint tendon.

33. a Inferior epigastric artery is lateral to the direct hernia.

34. b More than half are bilateral.

35. a Inguinal hernia.

36. a The presence of patent process vaginalis.

37. b Laparoscopic repair.

38. a Hernia repair as planned.

39. d Pubic tubercle.

40. b Adductor magnus.

41. a Femoral ring.

42. b Loss of fat.

43. a 4:1.

44. b Anaemia.

45. d 25%.

46. b Pre-operative hypotension.

47. a Omental patch closure and peritoneal lavage.

48. c Low serum fibrinogen level.

49. a Peptic ulcer disease.

50. d Site of bleeding.

51. a 8.

52. a It reduces the risk of active bleeding at the time of endoscopy.

53. b Posterior wall of the first part of the duodenum.

54. d Ulcer with a clean base.

55. c No therapeutic intervention.

56. b Antibiotics and interval cholecystectomy.

57. d The majority of patients present with abdominal pain, jaundice and fever.

58. b Percutaneous cholecystostomy.

59. c During the same admission.

60. b Adhesions.

61. a Incarceration of part of the circumference of the bowel.

62. b 3 mg/kg.

63. b Mesenteric ischaemia.

64. d Conservative management and barium enema after a few weeks before considering for surgery.

65. d Lower incidence of intra-abdominal abscess.

66. d All of the above.

67. a Ischaemic colitis.

68. a Sigmoid colon.

69. c X-ray abdomen.

70. d Computed tomography with rectal contrast.

71. a 0.1–0.5 mL/min.

72. b 1–1.5 mL/min.

73. d Upper gastrointestinal endoscopy.

74. b Rectal biopsy.

75. c Hypertrophic pyloric stenosis.

76. d Hypokalaemia, hyponatraemia, hypochloraemia.

77. **b** Metabolic alkalosis with paradoxical aciduria.

78. **b** Ultrasound.

79. **b** The majority of children with ileocolic intussusception present with intermittent abdominal pain, palpable mass and 'redcurrant jelly' stools.

80. **a** Patients who failed hydrostatic or pneumatic reduction.

81. **d** Intestinal obstruction.

82. **a** Tachycardia.

83. **a** 20 mL/kg bolus until signs of cardiovascular improvement.

84. **c** Meconium ileus.

85. **d** It can be carried out in A&E.

86. **a** Red cell count <100,000/mm^3.

87. **c** Stabilisation of the pelvis followed by laparotomy.

88. **a** 20 mmHg.

89. **a** Decreased central venous pressure.

90. **c** Increased preload.

91. **a** Increased lung compliance.

92. **a** Idiopathic.

93. **d** The greatest risk of post-operative pulmonary embolism is within 48 hours after surgery.

94. **a** Liver.

95. **b** 36 hours.

96. **c** Medical patients are at high risk compared to surgical patients.

97. a Factor V Leiden deficiency.

98. a Anti-cardiolipin antibodies.

99. b Hypokalaemia.

100. c Prophylactic platelet transfusion should be given due to the risk of bleeding.

101. b Deep vein thrombosis.

102. b Femoral vein thrombosis.

103. b Venography.

104. a Doppler ultrasound.

105. a Pulmonary embolism.

106. a Inhibition of factor Xa.

107. b Low molecular weight heparin.

108. d It can cause thrombocytopenia.

109. b Factor VII.

110. d It is associated with a lower incidence of type II heparin-induced thrombocytopenia (HIT).

111. d Renal failure.

112. d Patients at high risk of developing re-feeding syndrome should be started with full calorie and protein requirements on the first day.

113. d Maintenance of mean arterial pressure of 60 mmHg by non-adrenaline infusion.

114. d Dopexamine.

115. b Anti-thrombin.

116. c Increased glycogenolysis.

117. b Leukocytes, RBC, brain, kidney.

118. c Liver.

119. d All of the above.

120. d Cerebrovascular accident.

121. b Air embolism.

122. a Central line infection.

123. d Ilioinguinal nerve.

124. d Lumbar artery.

125. b Fascia covering the levator ani muscle.

126. d Nerve to the obturator internus.

127. b S 2, 3, 4.

128. a Inferior rectal nerve.

129. a Long-chain fatty acids.

130. a Purified blood from the placenta to the liver through the left branch of the portal vein.

131. a The phrenic nerve arises from the same segment of spinal cord as the supraclavicular nerves.

132. a Superior surface of the liver.

133. c Right free border of the lesser omentum.

134. b Tail of the pancreas.

135. d Anterior and posterior segments have their own blood supply separated by an avascular plane.

136. a Inguinal canal.

137. c Left testicular vein entering the renal vein at a right angle.

138. b Lower border of the 2nd thoracic vertebra.

139. c Posterior segment of the right upper lobe.

140. d All of the above.

141. d All of the above.

142. d All of the above.

143. d Cytoplasmic proteins.

144. a −2 to +2.

145. a Increased heart rate.

146. b Decreased stroke volume.

147. b Dobutamine.

148. a Factor VIII.

149. a 6 hours.

150. b 4 days.

151. a 25 mmHg.

152. a Tissue thromboplastin.

153. d Factor XII.

154. a −40 to −50°C.

155. a Bicarbonate ions.

156. b Curvilinear.

157. a The affinity of haemoglobin for O_2 following variation in $paCO_2$, H^+ ion and temperature.

158. c Absorption of potassium and bicarbonate ions.

159. a Ascending aorta just above the aortic valve leaflets.

160. a Diastole.

161. d Lower third of the thoracic oesophagus.

162. d Temperature.

163. a Hypoxia.

164. d Left ventricular failure.

165. d a and b.

166. b 0.2.

167. b 60 mmHg.

168. b Carboxyhaemoglobin.

169. d Consolidation.

170. c Both of the above.

171. c Liver.

172. a Observation.

173. d Small bowel.

174. a 20–24°C for 5 days.

175. b Prolonged QT interval.

176. a Congenital hypertrophic pyloric stenosis.

177. b Decreased K^+ in the urine.

178. a Hypokalaemia.

179. a 270 to 285.

180. b Dengue virus.

181. a At the end of expiration.

182. d Administration of fresh frozen plasma.

183. b Metabolic acidosis.

184. b Faeco-oral.

185. d Transversalis fascia.

186. d Ilioinguinal nerve.

187. a Surgery.

188. d Sigmoid colon.

189. a Bladder.

190. c Femoral hernia.

191. b Right apical lobe.

192. c Tracheobronchial injury.

193. d Intermittent positive pressure ventilation (IPPV).

194. d Pectoralis major.

195. a Intralesional injection of steroid.

196. c Presternal area.

197. a Malignant ulcer found on the scar of a burn.

198. c Local recurrence is common after excision.

199. b Liposarcoma.

200. c Embryonal rhabdomyosarcoma.

201. d S phase.

202. c G_1–S phase.

203. b Apoptosis.

204. c Hepatocellular carcinoma.

205. b Iodine-131.

206. c Carcinoma of the gallbladder.

207. c Carcinoma of the nasopharynx.

208. a Water.

209. a Ultrasonography.

210. b Metronidazole.

211. d Cyclin B.

212. b Hypercalcaemia.

213. c Ondansetron.

214. c Ovary.

215. b Parathyroid hormone related protein (PTHrP).

216. d Cobalt-60.

217. d G_2–M phase.

218. b Malignant melanoma.

219. c Cisplatinium.

220. b 10–14 mmHg.

221. a CO_2.

222. b Plasma imbibition.

223. c Full thickness grafts are mainly used for large areas of defect.

224. d Vasodilatation.

225. d Subcutaneous fasciectomy.

226. d Isotonic saline.

227. d Presence of blisters.

228. a Lactated Ringer's solution.

229. a 18%.

230. c Xenograft.

231. c 9%.

232. b 2nd degree.

233. b Wrist drop.

234. b Early skin grafting.

235. b High orchidectomy and retroperitoneal lymph node dissection.

236. c There are no germ cells.

237. c α-fetoprotein is markedly raised in all germ cell tumours.

238. a Testicular tumours.

239. a It remains in the scrotum.

240. c 12 months of age.

241. b Seminoma.

242. c Scrotum.

243. a Bleomycin, etoposide, cisplatin.

244. b Dysgerminoma.

245. b Para-aortic lymph nodes.

246. b Epididymo-orchitis.

247. b <10%.

248. a Increasing the velocity of venous blood.

249. c 3-fold.

250. c Serum transferrin.

251. c The risk of cancer reduces dramatically if it is corrected within six years.

252. b Seminoma.

253. a Motilin receptor agonist in the gastrointestinal tract.

254. b Dopamine receptor antagonist in the gastrointestinal tract.

255. c Malnutrition does not impair thermoregulation.

256. e All of the above.

257. a Patients with oesophageal obstruction secondary to malignancy.

258. c Patients who are likely to require nutritional support for less than 4 weeks should be considered for gastrostomy.

259. d Daily protein requirements are 2.0–2.5 g/kg/day.

260. b To avoid re-feeding problems, feed should be started at high volumes and reduced over a period of time.

261. e Iron and ferritin levels should be checked once every month.

262. d In patients following a recent uneventful laparotomy for left hemicolectomy.

263. c Cholestasis.

264. a High levels of carbohydrate increase CO_2 production.

265. b 1.0 kcal/mL energy.

266. e All of the above.

267. a Basal cell carcinoma.

268. a Distant metastases.

269. b 2 cm.

270. c Lateral surface of the thigh.

271. d 15 cm.

Index

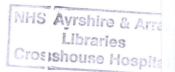